Praise for

ESSENTIALS OF PSYCHIATRIC DIAGNOSIS

"*Essentials of Psychiatric Diagnosis* is simply the best book I've read about how to accurately diagnose your patients. Frances's combination of vast experience, down-in-the-trenches common sense, and informed skepticism is unique. Whether you're a psychiatrist, psychologist, social worker, nurse, crisis counselor, or any other mental health professional, you should buy this book, read it cover to cover initially, and then keep it in your office to refer back to frequently. I'm glad this book had not been published before I wrote my book on the psychiatric interview, because the competition would have made me choose a different topic!"

—DANIEL J. CARLAT, MD, Department of Psychiatry, Tufts University School of Medicine; Founding Editor, *The Carlat Psychiatry Report*

"With his clinical expertise, leadership roles in prior DSM editions, and healthy skepticism about overdiagnosis and excessive medication, Frances has crafted a clinical gem. This clear and concise book describes a sequential assessment process and provides screening questions, easily remembered prototypic descriptions, differential diagnostic considerations, and cautionary notes about diagnostic traps. Frances recognizes the need for a diagnosis to guide intervention, while steering clear of diagnostic reification. All clinicians need this book for frequent reference, and it should be a required text in mental health training programs."

—JOHN F. CLARKIN, PhD, Personality Disorders Institute, New York Presbyterian Hospital; Department of Psychiatry, Weill Cornell Medical College

"This easy-to-read, commonsensical handbook guides mental health clinicians through the thicket of differential diagnosis in psychiatry. Frances—a thoughtful and effective critic of the excesses of DSM-5—shows where diagnosis is valid and essential, and where a premature diagnosis or a diagnostic fad has the potential to hurt patients. Everyone who uses diagnosis in daily practice will benefit from the down-to-earth wisdom of this book."

—JOEL PARIS, MD, Department of Psychiatry, McGill University, Canada

"This volume should head the list of user-friendly guides to psychiatric diagnosis. Frances draws on his considerable experience and contributions, such as heading the DSM-IV Task Force, to produce a work that will be indispensable for primary care clinicians and all professionals and students in mental health care. The guide contains screening questions, prototypic case descriptions, ICD-9-CM codes, and specific cautionary statements to reduce diagnostic inflation and raise concerns about aspects of DSM-5. The material is handled with sensitivity and compassion, with the patient's best interests always the central consideration. This book is a welcome arrival at a time when recent trends in diagnosis are increasingly attracting controversy. I will be using this excellent guide in my own work and will recommend it to my students and colleagues."

—ADRIAN WELLS, PhD, Division of Clinical Psychology, University of
    Manchester, United Kingdom

"A 'must have' for mental health professionals. Frances provides useful, easy-to-understand information about psychiatric diagnosis and coding for clinicians in all mental health disciplines."

—K. DAYLE JONES, PhD, LMHC, Mental Health Counseling Program,
    University of Central Florida

"Frances demonstrates an unusual ability to communicate the tacit knowledge of an expert into understandable concepts and ideas that will be appreciated by clinicians and students alike. Elegantly simple screening questions precede each disorder and cut through the diagnostic murk. Facilitating patient-centered care, teamwork, and collaboration, this is a comprehensive diagnostic resource for the whole treatment team."

—MARGARET (PEGGY) HALTER, PhD, APRN, Editor, *Foundations of
    Psychiatric Mental Health Nursing*; Associate Dean, Dwight Schar
    College of Nursing and Health Sciences, Ashland University

ESSENTIALS OF PSYCHIATRIC DIAGNOSIS

ESSENTIALS OF
PSYCHIATRIC DIAGNOSIS

Responding to the Challenge of DSM-5®

ALLEN FRANCES

THE GUILFORD PRESS
New York   London

© 2013 The Guilford Press
A Division of Guilford Publications, Inc.
72 Spring Street, New York, NY 10012
www.guilford.com

Printed in the United States of America

This book is printed on acid-free paper.

Last digit is print number: 9   8   7   6   5   4   3   2   1

The author has checked with sources believed to be reliable in his efforts to
provide information that is complete and generally in accord with the standards
of practice that are accepted at the time of publication. However, in view of the
possibility of human error or changes in behavioral, mental health, or medical
sciences, neither the author, nor the editor and publisher, nor any other party
who has been involved in the preparation or publication of this work warrants
that the information contained herein is in every respect accurate or complete,
and they are not responsible for any errors or omissions or the results obtained
from the use of such information. Readers are encouraged to confirm the
information contained in this book with other sources.

Library of Congress Cataloging-in-Publication Data

Frances, Allen, 1942–
   Essentials of psychiatric diagnosis: Responding to the challenge of DSM-5 /
Allen Frances.
      p. ; cm.
   Includes bibliographical references and index.
   ISBN 978-1-4625-1049-8 (pbk.: alk. paper)—ISBN 978-1-4625-1081-8 (hardcover:
alk. paper)
   I. Title.
   [DNLM: 1. Mental Disorders—diagnosis.   2. Diagnosis, Differential.
3. Mental Disorders—classification.   WM 141]
   RC473.D54
   616.89′075—dc23

                                                                    2013002075

DSM-5 is a registered trademark of the American Psychiatric Association.
The APA has not participated in the preparation of this book.

To my patients,
who taught me almost everything I know
about psychiatric diagnosis
and much of what I know about life

![] About the Author

Allen Frances, MD, is a clinician, educator, researcher, and leading authority on psychiatric diagnosis. He chaired the DSM-IV Task Force, was a member of the Task Force that prepared DSM-III-R, and wrote the final version of the Personality Disorders section in DSM-III. The author of several hundred papers and more than a dozen books, most recently *Saving Normal: An Insider's Revolt against Out-of-Control Psychiatric Diagnosis, DSM-5, Big Pharma, and the Medicalization of Ordinary Life,* Dr. Frances is Professor Emeritus and former Chair of the Department of Psychiatry and Behavioral Sciences at Duke University. He is an active blogger for *The Huffington Post, Psychology Today,* and *Education Update.*

Contents

CHAPTER 4

▣ Bipolar Disorders 49

CHAPTER 5

■ **Anxiety Disorders**   **61**

CHAPTER 8

■ Schizophrenia Spectrum and Other Psychotic Disorders 94

CHAPTER 11
■ Personality Disorders   130

CHAPTER 12
■ Impulse Control Disorders   138

CHAPTER 15

▪ Sexual and Gender Issues   **159**

CHAPTER 1

■ How to Use This Book

This book provides a concise and user-friendly guide to more accurate diagnosis and coding. It offers:

- One or more screening questions for each disorder. (Note that not every mental disorder in DSM-5 is covered in this book; I have omitted a few that do not seem useful.)
- Clear prototypal descriptions of these mental disorders, rather than complex and cumbersome criteria sets that are often ignored.
- The most crucial differential diagnoses that must be ruled out for each disorder.
- Diagnostic tips—everything I have learned through 40 years of seeing patients; supervising trainees; and preparing DSM-III, DSM-III-R, and DSM-IV.
- The required ICD-9-CM codes for each disorder.
- Cautions to reduce diagnostic inflation and counter the influence of fad diagnosing.
- Cautions on questionable aspects of DSM-5.

■ AUDIENCE

Essentials of Psychiatric Diagnosis is meant for everyone with an interest in psychiatric diagnosis. Practitioners from all the mental health disciplines and at all levels of experience should find valuable tips to aid them in arriving at the right diagnoses and codes. For beginning students and trainees, the book provides a manageable, but fairly comprehensive, introduction to the most important things worth knowing about psychiatric diagnosis. Test takers and board candidates will find it a valuable study guide. Harried primary care doctors (who do 80% of the prescribing of psychiatric medication)[1] will be directed toward an accurate diagnosis in the limited time they have with each patient. Seasoned clinicians may think they already know everything they need to know about diagnosis, but my experience suggests that most do not. I learned a lot in writing this book, and I doubt that there are many mental health workers who will not learn a lot in reading it. Last, but never least, are the patients and families who may find this a useful tool in the process of becoming more informed consumers. Patients have always been my teachers; it is nice to have the chance to return the favor. I have enjoyed writing this book and hope that all of its readers will enjoy using it.

Two notes on my use of pronouns are in order at the outset. First, although I use "you" to refer to "the clinician" in much of what follows, my intent is always to include patients and their families in my audience. Second, in referring to "the patient," I have generally tried to alternate between masculine and feminine pronouns, except in cases where patients with a particular diagnosis are almost all either male or female.

■ ORGANIZATION OF THE BOOK

Not every mental disorder included in DSM-5 is included in this book; I have omitted a few that simply do not seem useful. Morever, the sequence of mental disorders presented here differs sharply from their inconvenient organization in DSM-5. I have based their ordering roughly on their frequency of appearance in an average clinical practice and on the interetst typical clinicians and students will have in them. This helps to focus attention on the most important trees in the vast and dense forest of DSM mental disorders, and it highlights the issues that are most interesting and telling in differential diagnosis. A welcome bonus is that the book, so ordered, becomes a much more inviting and useful cover-to-cover read, not just a dry reference. The table of contents indicates the page on which each mental disorder is covered, along with its ICD-9-CM code.

Every disorder has its story to tell, and each illustrates the fascinating variety of human behavior in sickness and in health. Each chapter begins with a list of the disorders it covers. Within the chapters, the current official ICD-9-CM code is presented again with each disorder's main entry. By international treaty, all countries in the world use the codes of the *International Classification of Diseases* (ICD). The *Diagnostic and Statistical Manual of Mental Disorders* (DSM) codes are the same as, and are derived from, these ICD codes. They allow our reporting to meet treaty obligations and ensure that our statistics are compatible with those reported from the rest of the world.

Diagnostic Prototype versus Criteria for Diagnosis

The entry for each of the mental disorders begins with a screening question and a brief prototypal description. DSM-5 is such a large book in part because it contains sets of very detailed diagnostic criteria that define each diagnosis. The introduction of this method when DSM-III was published in 1980 was a great advance in the history of psychiatry because the careful use of criteria (especially in research and forensic environments) can lead to greatly enhanced reliability. Without criteria, psychiatric research would be impossible, and our field would lose credibility. But there is a hitch: Criteria sets are so cumbersome that most clinicians simply don't use them. Many say that they have committed the criteria sets to memory, but I know this is impossible. There are so many criteria for so many disorders that no one can possibly remember them. I have tested many very experienced and presumably expert diagnosticians on their recall of the specific items included in various criteria sets. They routinely fail, usually quite badly. Given the vicissitudes of memory, proper practice would be to look up the pertinent DSM sections before making a diagnosis, or to use a DSM checklist, but most busy clinicians do neither.

So I have taken an alternative approach in this book. Instead of offering diagnostic criteria that people won't remember, I provide a descriptive prototype for each diagnosis that captures its essence, hopefully in a more memorable way. This "prototypal method" is useful and convenient, and is the method almost all clinicians use anyway.[2] But it also has clear limitations. More precise diagnosis (using explicit and detailed diagnostic criteria, and perhaps semistructured interviews) is clearly preferable for situations where more time is available and when establishing reliability is of paramount importance—for example, in research studies, in forensic proceedings, in disability determinations, when the diagnosis is particularly unclear, or when treatment based on a prior diagnosis has failed.[3]

Differential Diagnosis and Diagnostic Tips

Following each prototypic description, there is a comprehensive differential diagnosis listing the conditions that need to be ruled out. Diagnostic tips specific to each diagnosis are provided. Whenever the differential diagnosis is difficult, you will find it useful to go back and forth between the likely contenders as you consider where your patient fits best. If there is insufficient information to permit you to choose between them, or if neither really fits well, feel comfortable being tentative with the best "Unspecified" choice (see below).

Index of Disorders by Symptoms

The Index of Disorders by Symptoms allows you to determine which mental disorders should be considered for each presenting symptom. Checking this is a useful way to ensure that you are not missing any of the possibilities.

■ CONTAINING DIAGNOSTIC INFLATION AND AVOIDING FADS

Retrospective epidemiological studies report that 20% of the general population qualifies for a current psychiatric diagnosis and 50% for a lifetime one.[4] Prospective epidemiological studies double these rates and suggest that mental disorder is becoming virtually ubiquitous.[5, 6] During the past 20 years, we have experienced three unanticipated fads partly precipitated by DSM-IV: a 20-fold increase in Autism Spectrum Disorder,[7] a tripling of Attention-Deficit/Hyperactivity Disorder (ADHD),[8] and a doubling of Bipolar Disorders.[9] The most dangerous fad is a 40-fold increase in childhood Bipolar Disorders,[10] stimulated, not by DSM-IV, but instead by reckless and misleading drug company marketing. Twenty percent of the U.S. population[11] is taking a psychotropic drug; 7% is addicted to one; and overdoses with legal drugs now cause more emergency room visits than overdoses with illegal drugs.[12, 13]

I don't think we are experiencing a real epidemic of increased mental disorders; instead, we are in the midst of an epidemic of careless diagnosis and loose prescription habits. Very small changes in how disorders are defined and in how the diagnostic criteria are applied can result in enormous changes in the reported rates of disorders and in the use of medications. Part of my goal in this book is to help correct diagnostic inflation and curtail or prevent fads. Whenever appropriate, I provide cautions and recommendations on how to avoid the loose diagnostic practice that leads to overdiagnosis. The wise clinician is always cautious and goes against fads rather than joining them. If everyone suddenly seems to have a diagnosis *du jour,* most probably don't.

▪ PROBLEMS WITH DSM-5

DSM-5 suffers from the unfortunate combination of unrealistically lofty ambitions and sloppy methodology.[14] Its optimistic hope was to create a paradigm-shifting advance in psychiatry; instead, the sad result is a manual that is not safe and not scientifically sound.[15] For example, it has introduced three new disorders that are at the fuzzy boundary with normality: Binge-Eating Disorder, Mild Neurocognitive Disorder, and Disruptive Mood Dysregulation Disorder. Unless these diagnoses are used with restraint, millions of essentially normal people will be mislabeled and subjected to potentially harmful treatment and unnecessary stigma. DSM-5 has also lowered the requirements for diagnosing existing disorders. For example, 2 weeks of normal grief have been turned into Major Depressive Disorder. The criteria for adult ADHD have been loosened, making it easily confused with normal distractibility and facilitating the illegal misuse of prescription stimulants for performance enhancement or recreational purposes. DSM-5 has collapsed early Substance Abuse and end-stage Substance Dependence (addiction) into one category, confusing their very different courses and treatment needs and creating unnecessary stigma.[16]

None of these changes was based on a solid scientific foundation; none has been tested sufficiently; none has any proven relation to effective treatment; and all are subject to grave misuse. For example, Disruptive Mood Dysregulation Disorder is included in DSM-5, despite its having been studied by just one research group for only 6 years. A petition by 51 mental health associations that the DSM-5 changes be reviewed by independent experts in evidence-based medicine was rejected without explanation.[17] DSM-5 has thus opened the floodgates to worsened diagnostic inflation and to excessive medication use.

CAUTION Boxes

My advice is to beware of changes introduced by DSM-5 that encourage diagnostic inflation. To aid clinicians in avoiding such inflation, I have discussed problematic DSM-5 disorders in Caution boxes within relevant sections. The boxes include explanations of why I think these specific diagnoses should be used rarely, if at all. Caution boxes also appear following the diagnostic prototypes for those established disorders most likely to be misdiagnosed if the lowered DSM-5 thresholds are used.

Be mindful that not all symptoms and problems in living are caused by mental disorders, and that mislabeling can be extremely harmful to those mislabeled. In judgment call situations, it is always much safer and more accurate to underdiagnose than to overdiagnose. It is easy enough to add a diagnosis when time and experience prove it to be appropriate, but once a misdiagnosis is made, it takes on a life of its own and is very hard to unmake. In the rest of this chapter, I offer clinicians some practical guidelines for reaching accurate diagnoses.

■ THE DIAGNOSTIC INTERVIEW

The Relationship Comes First

An accurate diagnosis comes from a collaborative effort with a patient. It is both the product of that good relationship and one of the best ways of promoting it. The first interview is a challenging moment, risky but potentially magical. Great things can happen if a good relationship is forged and the right diagnosis is made. But if you fail to hit it off well in the first visit, the person may never come back for a second. And the patient doesn't always make it easy. It is likely that you are meeting him on one of the worst days of his life. People often wait until their suffering is so desperate that it finally outweighs the fear, mistrust, or embarrassment that previously prevented them from seeking help. For you, a new patient may be just the eighth patient you see in a long and hectic work day. For this patient, the encounter is often freighted with expectations that are exaggerated for good or for bad. Every diagnostic evaluation is important for the patient, and it should be for you too. The focus, first and always, should be on the patient's need to be heard and understood; this must trump all else.

Make Diagnosis a Team Effort

Make the search for the diagnosis a joint project that displays your empathy, not a dry affair that feels invasive—and always provide information and education. The patient should walk out feeling both understood and enlightened. Never forget that this evaluation may be a crucial tipping point that can change the patient's entire future.

Maintain Balance in the First Moments

There are two opposite types of risk that occur in the first moments of the first interview. Many clinicians prematurely jump to diagnostic conclusions based on very limited data and stay stuck on incorrect first impressions, blinded to subsequent contradictory facts. At the other extreme are those who focus too slowly, missing the amazingly rich information that immediately pours forth on the first meeting with a patient. Patients come in primed to convey a great deal to you, intentionally and unintentionally, through words and demeanor. Maintain balance—be extra alert in those first few minutes, but don't jump quickly to diagnostic conclusions.

Balance Open-Ended with Checklist Questions

Until DSM-III, training in interviewing skills emphasized the importance of giving the patient the widest freedom of expression. This was extremely useful in bringing out what was most individual in each person's presentation, but the lack of structure and specific questioning led to very poor diagnostic reliability. Clinicians can agree on diagnosis only if they gather equivalent information and are working off the same database. The desire to achieve reliability and efficiency has led clinicians at some centers to go very far in the opposite direction: They do closed-ended, "laundry list" interviews focused only on getting yes–no answers to questions exclusively based on DSM criteria. Carried to extremes, both approaches lose the patient—the former to idiosyncratic free form, the latter to narrow reductionism. Let your patients reveal themselves spontaneously, but also manage to ask the questions that need to be asked.

Use Screening Questions to Hone in on the Diagnosis

The surest way toward a reliable, accurate, and comprehensive diagnosis is a semistructured interview that combines a wide range of open-ended and closed-ended questions. However, this takes hours to perform and is possible only in highly specialized research or forensic situations, where time is no object and reliability is all-important. The everyday clinical interview necessarily requires shortcuts; you can't ask every question about every disorder. After listening carefully to the patient's presenting problems, you must select which branch of the diagnostic tree to climb first. Place the symptoms among the most pertinent of the broad categories (e.g., Depressive Disorders, Bipolar Disorders, Anxiety Disorders, Obsessive–Compulsive Disorder [OCD], Psychotic Disorders, Substance-Related Disorders, etc.). Then ask screening questions (provided for each disorder) to start narrowing down to the particular diagnostic prototype that best fits the patient. Before feeling comfortable with your diagnosis, make sure you explore with the patient the alternative possibilities covered in the differential diagnosis section for that disorder. I'll be giving diagnostic tips that will help you along the way. Always check for the role of medicines, other substances, and medical illnesses in everyone you evaluate.

Remember the Significance of Clinical Significance

Psychiatric symptoms are fairly ubiquitous in the general population. Most normal people have at least one, and many have a few. When present in isolation, a single symptom (or even a few) do not by themselves constitute psychiatric illness. Two additional conditions must also be met before symptoms can be considered mental disorder. **First**, they have to cluster in a characteristic way. Isolated symptoms of depression, anxiety, insomnia, memory difficulties, attention problems, and so forth are never by themselves sufficient to justify a diagnosis. **Second**, the symptoms must cause clinically significant distress or clinically significant impairment in social or occupational functioning. This caveat is so important that it is a central and essential aspect of the differential diagnosis for most of the psychiatric disorders. Keep always in mind that it is never enough to identify symptoms; they must also create serious and persistent problems.

Conduct a Risk–Benefit Analysis

In toss-up situations, weigh the pluses and minuses of giving the diagnosis. The basic question boils down to "Is this diagnosis more likely to help or more likely to hurt?" All else being equal when decisions could go either way, it makes sense to make a diagnosis when it has a recommended treatment that has been proven safe and effective—but to withhold a questionable diagnosis if there is no proven treatment or if the available treatment has potentially dangerous side effects. Stepped diagnosis (see below) provides time for the clinical picture to declare itself and for you to get a deeper understanding of it.

Don't Misunderstand Comorbidity

In order to facilitate reliability, DSM is a splitter's (not a lumper's) system; the diagnostic pie has been cut into many very small slices. Many patients present with more than one cluster of symptoms and require more than one diagnosis. Noting all the pertinent diagnoses adds diagnostic precision and provides a more rounded view of the person. But having more than one disorder doesn't mean that each is independent of one another, or that they require separate treatments. The DSM mental disorders are no more than descriptive syndromes; they are not necessarily discrete diseases. The multiple diagnoses may reflect one underlying etiology and may respond to one treatment. For example, Panic Disorder and Generalized Anxiety Disorder may be just two faces of the same tendency toward problems with anxiety. It is useful to have separate categories for each because some people have only panic symptoms and others only generalized anxiety symptoms. Having separate categories adds information and precision, but should not imply separate causalities or need for separate treatments. Misunderstanding comorbidity can lead to harmful polypharmacy if a clinician believes incorrectly that each mental disorder necessarily requires its own treatment.

Be Patient

With some people, things are so clear-cut that the diagnosis jumps out in 5 minutes. But with others, it may take 5 hours. With still others, it may require 5 months or even 5 years. Diagnostic impressions are useful hypotheses to be tested, not blinders that can cause you to miss newer information or the bigger picture. If you rush into a diagnosis, serious mistakes can be made.

Don't Be Ashamed to Use
the "Unspecified" Categories

How simple it would be if our patients' symptoms conformed closely with the neat little packages that are contained in the DSM definitions. But real life is always so much more complicated than what is written down on paper. Psychiatric presentations are heterogeneous and overlapping and often have the fuzziest of boundaries. Lots of times, someone has symptoms that bespeak the presence of a mental disorder, but that don't fall precisely within the boundaries of any one of the named DSM categories. This is the reason why the many "Unspecified" categories are sprinkled so liberally throughout DSM-5. These categories provide indispensable placeholders when patients definitely need a diagnosis, but don't fit existing molds. Without them, the diversity of human suffering would require that we include an ever-expanding list of additional new mental disorders—thus risking overdiagnosis and burying the system in unmanageable complexity.

Psychiatry has many shades of gray that are lost with black-and-white thinking. Using the Unspecified label reflects and announces that there is an appreciable level of diagnostic uncertainty—a useful thing when the simple, fast answer is so often wrong and harmful. Uncertainty can arise when there is insufficient information, or when a patient has an atypical or subthreshold presentation, or when it is unclear whether substances or medical illnesses are causing the symptoms. The Unspecified designation implies that we will need to extend the evaluation and learn much more before committing ourselves. Admitting uncertainty is a good first step to accurate diagnosis. Pseudoprecision is no precision, and premature certainty brings no certainty; instead, both lead to the dangerous unintended consequences of unnecessary stigma and excessive medication treatment.

Suppose that a patient has an apparent depression, but it is not yet clear whether the symptoms constitute a primary Depressive Disorder, are secondary to alcohol use or to a medical illness, are medication side effects, or are some combination of these. Until the picture comes into clearer focus, Unspecified Depressive Disorder is just the ticket. Or suppose that a teenager presents with a first onset of psychotic symptoms, and it is too soon to tell whether this is a Bipolar Disorder, Brief Psychotic Disorder, or the result of multiple secret LSD trips. Stick with Unspecified Psychotic Disorder until time (ideally) tells all. Don't "ready, fire, aim."

There is one important disclaimer. Wonderful and necessary as the Unspecified categories are in clinical practice, they are unreliable and completely useless in forensic proceedings and should never be taken seriously if offered as expert testimony. Forensic work requires a much higher degree of precision and agreement than can ever be afforded by the Unspecified diagnoses.

Be Cautious about "Other" Diagnoses

DSM-5 has introduced a new convention that I consider risky. For many categories, the clinician can code "Other"—as in Other Psychotic Disorder, Other Mood Disorder, Other Anxiety Disorder, or Other Paraphilic Disorder. I object to this because it provides a back-door way to diagnose proposed conditions that have been explicitly rejected by DSM-5 or relegated to Section 3, for disorders requiring further study, such as Attenuated Psychosis Syndrome, Mixed Anxiety/Depression, Coercive Paraphilia, Hebephilia, Internet Addiction, Sex Addiction, and so forth. These have all been rejected or kept at arm's length for very good reasons and should not be used casually in clinical or forensic practice. For the sake of consistency, I sometimes include codes for the Other categories, but I omit them when they are particularly likely to be misused.

Constantly Test Your Subjective Judgments

There are no biological tests in psychiatry, and (with the exception of tests for dementia) none are in the pipeline for at least the next decade. Psychiatric diagnosis depends completely on subjective judgments that are necessarily fallible, should always be tentative, and must constantly be tested as you know the patient better and see how the course evolves. The more information the better, especially since people aren't always the most accurate reporters about themselves. Whenever possible, speak with family members and other informants, and also get records (both medical records and records of any previous psychiatric or other mental health treatments). You shouldn't necessarily believe past diagnoses—people change, and diagnostic errors are frequent—but you should take them into account. And whenever treatment isn't working, always reconsider the diagnosis.

Always Document Your Thinking

By itself, a diagnosis is just a naked label. It will help your clinical think-ing and your longitudinal follow-up (and protect you from malpractice suits) if you also provide a clear rationale for your conclusions as you are forming them. What are the factors in the patient's current presentation, personal history, course, family history, and previous treatment response that most guided your thinking? What are the unanswered questions and areas of continuing uncertainty? What will you be looking for in future visits? Good documentation is a sign of, and also a guide to, good diag-nostic practice.

Remember That the Stakes Are High

Done well, psychiatric diagnosis leads to appropriate treatment and a good chance for cure or at least substantial improvement. Done poorly, psychiatric diagnosis leads to a nightmare of harmful treatments, unnec-essary stigma, missed opportunities, reduced expectations, and negative self-fulfilling prophecies. It is worth the time and effort to become really good at psychiatric diagnosis. Being a competent diagnostician won't guarantee that you are a complete clinician, but it is impossible to be even a satisfactory clinician without good diagnostic skills.

■ STEPPED DIAGNOSIS

The biggest single cause of inaccurate diagnosis is jumping to premature conclusions. The best guarantee of accuracy and safety is "stepped diag-nosis." When the appropriate diagnosis is completely obvious and easily agreed upon, you can make it quickly and confidently. This is particu-larly true for the classic presentations of the more severe disorders. But a stepped approach to diagnosis is more accurate and efficient for people who present with milder or ambiguous symptoms, or who have too short a history to provide a basis for future prediction. Rashly attempting quick closure is likely to be premature, mistaken, and harmful.

Step 1: Engage in Watchful Waiting

As noted earlier, many people come for their first visit when symptoms are at their highest pitch. They may look quite different, and often seem much less troubled, on repeat visits. An accurate diagnosis is often impossible if you have just one unrepresentative snapshot of a person's entire life. Except in the clearest cases, always underdiagnose (or don't diagnose at all) during early visits.

Step 2: Make Sure the Symptoms Are Severe and Persistent Enough to Count

Psychiatric symptoms are widely distributed in the general population. Sadness, anxiety, trouble sleeping, fatigue, somatic symptoms—all are part of the everyday experience of living. It is only when symptoms are grouped together in a recognized pattern, persist over time, and cause clinically significant distress or impairment that a diagnosis of mental disorder is warranted.

Step 3: Educate, Normalize, Reassure

It is useful for people to know that their symptoms may turn out to be normal, expectable, and transient reactions to life's stresses and disappointments. Education and reassurance can often go a long way toward promoting rapid symptom reduction and providing a clearer diagnostic picture. Of course, the normalization and reassurance must be realistic and also must not minimize the magnitude of real problems.

Step 4: Rule Out the Role of Substances

Always be sure to consider whether substance use or a medication side effect is the possible cause of the patient's presentation. Psychiatric symptoms are a final common pathway with many possible causes. Substance Abuse and Dependence can warp functioning in a way that faithfully mimics many of the mental disorders. And people are often reluctant to admit they have a substance use problem; careful questioning and timely laboratory testing may be necessary. Also remember that medications cause psychiatric side effects—particularly in the elderly, in persons who are taking many different medicines (which may interact with one another), and in persons who are taking one or more medicines in high doses.

Step 5: Rule Out the Role of Medical Illness

Especially in the elderly, always consider neurological or other medical illness as a possible cause of the psychiatric problems. It is not a bad idea to recommend a medical evaluation and appropriate laboratory testing for everyone as a routine part of the diagnostic process.

Step 6: Rule Out Bipolar and Depressive Disorders

Bipolar and Depressive Disorders are common, are heterogeneous, and can include a wide variety of symptoms seen in many other conditions (e.g., anxiety; eating, sleeping, and/or sexual problems; decrements in cognitive function; hallucinations and delusions; personality changes; somatic distress; and so on). Always consider Bipolar and Depressive Disorders first before making another diagnosis.

■ A DOZEN GENERAL TIPS

The 12 tips below are meant to set the stage for accurate and safe diagnosis. Much more specific tips are provided for each disorder in subsequent chapters.

1. **Hippocrates said that knowing the patient is just as important as knowing the disease.** Don't get so caught up in the details of the symptoms that you miss the context in which they occur.
2. **Take the time and make the effort.** It takes time to make the right diagnosis—adequate time for each interview, and often multiple interviews over time to see how things are evolving.
3. **If you hear hoofbeats on Broadway, think horses, not zebras!** When in doubt, go with the odds. Like exotic animals, exotic diagnoses may be fun to think about, but you almost never see them in real life. Stick with the more common diagnoses and you will rarely go wrong.
4. **Get all the information you can.** No one source is ever complete.

Triangulation of data from multiple information sources leads to a more reliable diagnosis.

5. **Consider previous diagnoses, but don't blindly believe them.** As noted earlier, incorrect diagnoses tend to have a long half-life and unfortunate staying power. Always do your own careful evaluation of the person's entire longitudinal course.

6. **Constantly revisit the diagnosis.** This is especially true when someone is not benefiting from a treatment that is based on the diagnosis. Clinicians can get tunnel vision once they've fixed on a diagnosis, and may become blinded to contradictory data.

7. **Children and teenagers are especially hard to diagnose.** They have a short track record, mature at varying rates, may be using drugs or alcohol, and are reactive to family and environmental stresses. The initial diagnosis is likely to be unstable and inappropriate.

8. **The elderly are also hard to diagnose.** Their psychiatric symptoms may be caused by neurological or other medical illness, and they are prone to drug side effects, interactions, and overdoses.

9. **The less severe the presentation, the more difficult it is to diagnose.** There is no bright line demarcating the very heavily populated boundary between mental disorder and normality. Milder problems often resolve spontaneously with time and without need for diagnosis or treatment.

10. **When you are in doubt, it is safer and more accurate to underdiagnose.** It's easier to step up to a more severe diagnosis than to step down from it.

11. **Accurate diagnosis can bring great benefits; inaccurate diagnosis can bring disaster.**

12. **Always remember the other enduring dictum from Hippocrates: "First, do no harm."**

■ REFERENCES

1. Mark TL et al. (2009): Datapoints: Psychotropic drug prescriptions by medical specialty. *Psychiatric Services, 9*(60), 1167, and Healthcare Business of Thomson Reuters.
2. Westen D (2012): Prototype diagnosis of psychiatric syndromes. *World Psychiatry, 11*(1), 16–21.

3. Frances A (2012): Prototypal diagnosis: Will this relic from the past become the wave of the future? *World Psychiatry, 11*(1), 26.
4. Kessler RC et al. (2005): Lifetime prevalence and age-of-onset distributions of DSM-IV disorders in the National Comorbidity Survey Replication. *Archives of General Psychiatry, 62*(6), 593–602.
5. Moffitt TE et al. (2010): How common are common mental disorders?: Evidence that lifetime prevalence rates are doubled by prospective versus retrospective ascertainment. *Psychological Medicine, 40*(6), 899–909.
6. Copeland W et al. (2011): Cumulative prevalence of psychiatric disorders by young adulthood: A prospective cohort analysis from the Great Smoky Mountains Study. *Journal of the American Academy of Child and Adolescent Psychiatry, 50*(3), 252–261.
7. Centers for Disease Control and Prevention (2012): CDC estimates 1 in 88 children in United States has been identified as having an Autism Spectrum Disorder (accessed October 8, 2012). *www.cdc.gov/media/releases/2012/p0329_autism_disorder.html*
8. Bloom B et al. (2011): Summary health statistics for U.S. children: National Health Interview Survey, 2010. *Vital Health Statistics, 10*(250). *www.cdc.gov/nchs/data/series/sr_10/sr10_250.pdf*
9. Ketter TA (2010): Diagnostic features, prevalence, and impact of bipolar disorder. *Journal of Clinical Psychiatry, 71*(6), e14.
10. Moreno C et al. (2007): National trends in the outpatient diagnosis and treatment of bipolar disorder in youth. *Archives of General Psychiatry, 64*, 1032–1039.
11. Medco Health Solutions (2011): *America's state of mind.* St. Louis, MO: Author.
12. Centers for Disease Control and Prevention (2011): Prescription painkiller overdoses at epidemic levels. *www.cdc.gov/media/releases/2011/p1101_flu_pain_killer_overdose.html*
13. Murphy K (2012, April 7): A fog of drugs and war. *Los Angeles Times* (accessed September 16, 2012). *http://articles.latimes.com/2012/apr/07/nation/la-na-army-medication-20120408*
14. Frances A (2009): A warning sign on the road to DSM-V: Beware of its unintended consequences. *Psychiatric Times, 26*(8), 1–4.
15. Frances A (2010): The first draft of DSM-V. *British Medical Journal, 340*, c1168.
16. Frances A (2009): Whither DSM-V? *British Journal of Psychiatry, 195*(5), 391–392.
17. Division 32 Committee on DSM-5 (2012): The open letter to DSM-5 Task Force (accessed October 8, 2012). *http://dsm5-reform.com/the-open-letter-to-dsm-5-task-force*

CHAPTER 2

■ Disorders Usually First Diagnosed in Childhood and Adolescence

IN THIS CHAPTER:

- ■ Attention-Deficit/Hyperactivity Disorder
- ■ CAUTION: ADHD and Age
- ■ Conduct Disorder and Oppositional Defiant Disorder
  - • Conduct Disorder
  - • Oppositional Defiant Disorder
  - • Unspecified Disruptive Behavior Disorder
- ■ Autism Spectrum Disorder
- ■ Separation Anxiety Disorder
- ■ Intellectual Developmental Disorder
- ■ Learning Disorder
- ■ Feeding Disorders
  - • Pica
  - • Rumination Disorder
- ■ Elimination Disorders
  - • Encopresis With Constipation and Overflow Incontinence
  - • Encopresis Without Constipation and Overflow Incontinence
  - • Enuresis

■ ATTENTION-DEFICIT/HYPERACTIVITY DISORDER

314.01 Attention-Deficit/Hyperactivity Disorder, Predominantly Hyperactive–Impulsive

314.00 Attention-Deficit/Hyperactivity Disorder, Predominantly Inattentive

314.01 Attention-Deficit/Hyperactivity Disorder, Combined

314.9 Unspecified Attention-Deficit/Hyperactivity Disorder

Screening Question

If patient is a child: "Is your child restless, always on the go, impulsive, and/or unable to focus on the task at hand?"

If patient is an adult: "Have hyperactivity and distractibility been problems for you, going as far back as you can remember?"

Diagnostic Prototype

Some children with ADHD (particularly boys) are just hyperactive and impulsive. Others (particularly girls) are just inattentive. Most show combinations of both, with the overactivity gradually becoming less of a problem as they grow up. About two-thirds continue to have symptoms as adults, usually in attenuated form. The symptoms must be inherent in the individual and seen in multiple settings (e.g., home, school, clinician's office); they should not just be reactions to a particular situation.

Hyperactivity–Impulsivity

The child is hectic, driven, impatient, jumpy, and all over the place—a kind of perpetual-motion machine. He is living at fast-forward pace—a hummingbird who is almost never still, quiet, relaxed, or at peace. Should other people happen to get in the way, they are banged into, run over, intruded upon, and interrupted, often loudly and insensitively. There are quick shifts from one activity to another without ever completing the previous task. It is seemingly impossible to postpone gratification or resist temptation. Decisions are made quickly and impulsively, without sufficient planning, thought, or consideration of risks or consequences.

Inattention

The child can't concentrate; she is easily distracted, absent-minded, and forgetful. She is usually late, misses deadlines, is careless, is mistake-prone, and is always losing her stuff. Her work is messy, disorganized, and far below her capacity.

CAUTION: ADHD and Age

Age of Onset

DSM-5 makes the mistake of allowing ADHD to have an initial onset as late as age 12. Instead, I would suggest you not make the diagnosis unless clear, strong signs of ADHD have appeared by age 7 or earlier. Kids with reliably diagnosable ADHD are pretty much born with the problems and show them early. Allowing later onset further confuses ADHD with the many other psychiatric causes of hyperactivity, impulsivity, and distractibility. Later onsets are likely to have other causes. Be especially cautious about diagnosing ADHD for the first time in an adult, since there is a high probability that the symptoms are within normal limits or due to something else and stimulant medication may be sought for recreation, performance enhancement, or resale. Stepped diagnosis is a step in the right direction.

Adult ADHD

DSM-5 has reduced the symptom requirement for adult ADHD and has also loosened the required age of onset. These changes may encourage the fad diagnosis of adult ADHD, leading to marked overprescription of stimulant medication, often for performance enhancement or recreation. Don't join the fad. Before making the diagnosis, ensure that the symptoms go back to early childhood, are not just associated features of another psychiatric disorder, and are so severe as to warrant being considered a mental disorder. Also beware of possible Malingering to obtain medication for improper use or resale.

Differential Diagnosis: Rule These Conditions Out

- **Normal immaturity.** What is developmentally appropriate and completely normal at 4 may be ADHD at 7.
- **Individual difference.** There is no clinically significant impairment.
- **Oppositional Defiant Disorder (ODD).** The behaviors arise from willful refusal to comply with structure or authority.

- **Conduct Disorder.** There is a pattern of severe violation of rules.
- **Intellectual Developmental Disorder.** The child seems inattentive or disorganized only because he can't keep up with the work.
- **Adjustment Disorder.** Symptoms are responses to a chaotic school environment, family stress, or change in life circumstances.
- **Other mental disorder.** Remember that hyperactivity, impulsivity, and inattentiveness are common symptoms across all of psychiatry (substance use, mania, dementia, etc., etc.).
- **Malingering.** The patient wants a prescription for stimulant drugs for performance enhancement, recreation, or resale.

Diagnostic Tips

- **Rising prevalence.** ADHD rates have tripled in recent years; it is now diagnosed in up to an astounding 10% of all kids. Some of this comes from better identification of previously missed cases, but there is much overdiagnosis—under pressure from drug company marketing, and because ADHD is often a prerequisite for receiving school services and extra time for test taking.
- **Developmental differences.** ADHD is also overdiagnosed because normal and expectable individual and developmental differences have been medicalized and treated excessively with pills. The most striking example is that being born in December rather than January is a strong risk factor for ADHD when a January 1 birthday is the cutoff for grade assignment. The younger, less mature children in class (particularly boys) are at serious risk for ADHD misdiagnosis and unnecessary medicine.
- **Nonspecificity of ADHD symptoms.** Hyperactivity, impulsivity, and distractibility are all very widely distributed in the normal population and are symptoms of many psychiatric disorders.
- **Requirements other than presence of symptoms.** Remember that it is not enough that symptoms be present. It is also necessary for the symptoms to have early onset; to be developmentally inappropriate and persistent; to be present in more than one setting (e.g., school and home); to cause significant functional problems or distress; and not to be due to any other psychiatric disorder. Attending to all these requirements will reduce careless overdiagnosis of ADHD.
- **Stepped diagnosis.** In the case of ADHD, this includes watchful wait-

ing, parent training, recalibration of perfectionistic parent and teacher expectations, and environmental manipulations.

• **Persistence of symptoms.** The ADHD behaviors should have been present for at least 6–12 months. Given time, kids will often outgrow a developmental phase or stressful time in their lives.

• **Role of the environment.** Overdiagnosis of ADHD in children is particularly likely if parents and/or teachers are stressed and overworked; if adults expect too much; and/or if there is a disruptive home or classroom environment.

• **Informants.** Information should come from as many sources as possible, to tease out the degree to which the problem is in the environment rather than in the child.

• **Possible role of substance use.** Substances can cause all the symptoms of ADHD. Be especially suspicious if problems have a late onset (after or around the time of puberty).

• **Pill diversion.** There is a large market for stimulants diverted away from their intended prescribed use and instead sold or given away, so that others can use them for recreation or performance enhancement. Thirty percent of college students and 10% of high school students have inappropriately obtained stimulant drugs in this way.

■ CONDUCT DISORDER AND OPPOSITIONAL DEFIANT DISORDER

312.81 Conduct Disorder, Childhood-Onset Type
312.82 Conduct Disorder, Adolescent-Onset Type
312.89 Conduct Disorder, Unspecified Onset

Screening Question

"Does your child get into a lot of trouble?"

Diagnostic Prototype

The child shows little or no respect for his (much more rarely, her) parents, the law, or the rights or feelings of others. This results in a persistent pattern of varied and repeated misbehaviors that involve physical and verbal aggression; the theft or destruction of property; deception, cheating, and manipulation; and the violation of rules and laws. He disrupts the family, gets into trouble at school, and may have periodic contacts with the juvenile justice system. The problems are always "someone else's fault."

Differential Diagnosis: Rule These Conditions Out

- **No mental disorder.** The misbehaviors are not severe and do not cause clinically significant impairment.
- **Adjustment Disorder.** The bad conduct does not exceed the cultural norms in the kid's environment, or he is responding to a chaotic or abusive family situation.
- **Oppositional Defiant Disorder.** ODD also has a pattern of defiance to authority, but without the severe and pervasive lack of respect for the law and the rights of others.
- **Substance Use Disorders.** Misbehaviors occur only in relation to Substance Intoxication or Dependence.
- **Attention-Deficit/Hyperactivity Disorder.** ADHD can cause behavioral scrapes, but not of the same magnitude and pervasiveness.
- **Bipolar or Depressive Disorders.** Misbehavior occurs in the context of clear depressive or manic symptoms.
- **Child or Adolescent Antisocial Behavior.** Any one isolated act of misbehavior, however severe, does not constitute a mental disorder. Code it V71.02.

Diagnostic Tips

- **The child or the environment?** The diagnosis of Conduct Disorder brings up the difficult conundrum of how best to separate psychiatric disorder from social or family problems.
  - ○ **Contribution from the child.** The concept of mental disorder implies that the repetitive misbehaviors arise from problems within the individual and are not just the result of being brought up in a chaotic and hostile environment where misbehavior is a cultural norm. The DSM definition of Conduct Disorder doesn't help much; it rests on a strictly descriptive listing of bad behaviors, and it makes no causal inferences concerning the relative contribution arising from the child versus the environment.

- ○ **Contribution from the setting.** Be on the cautious side before applying the psychiatric term Conduct Disorder to kids growing up in impossible environments. The diagnosis may focus too much attention on the child's contribution, and too little on the need to do everything possible to provide a more wholesome setting. When in doubt, diagnose Adjustment Disorder, not Conduct Disorder.

- **The child or the substance?** A similar cause-and-effect conundrum comes from the fact that early Substance Abuse is a manifestation of Conduct Disorder, but also is itself a direct cause of misbehavior. What was believed to be Conduct Disorder may disappear altogether if the substance problem is successfully addressed.

- **Risk factors.** The earlier the bad behavior, and the greater its aggressiveness and severity, the more likely it is to persist into adulthood. The less severe the behavior and the later its onset, the more likely it is to be transient and due to substance use, peer pressure, developmental issues, and/or family troubles.

- **Rates of conversion.** About one-third of kids with Conduct Disorder persist in their misbehaviors and go on to qualify as adults for the diagnosis of Antisocial Personality Disorder. Everyone with adult Antisocial Personality Disorder must have evidence of childhood Conduct Disorder. Were this not required, virtually all criminals would be labeled as having a mental disorder, and the term would lose all meaning.

- **Relation to ODD.** Conduct Disorder and ODD represent a severity continuum of bad behavior, with no clear boundary separating the two diagnoses. In a doubtful case, give the child the benefit of the doubt and go with the less severe diagnosis of ODD— especially if the child is growing up in a stressful and tough environment.

313.81 Oppositional Defiant Disorder

Screening Question

"Do you have a lot of power struggles with your child?"

Diagnostic Prototype

The child is a pain to the parent—angry most of the time, argumentative, quick to say "No!" to everything, and unwilling to obey rules or follow instructions. Easily annoyed, he (sometimes she) also seems to delight in being annoying. Every limit is tested; everything is someone else's fault. The child manages to feel forever misunderstood and put upon.

Differential Diagnosis: Rule These Conditions Out

- **Developmentally normal willfulness.** Part of growing up is establishing independence and a separate identity.
- **Parent–Child Relational Problem.** This is not considered a mental disorder in either player. Code it V61.20.
- **Adjustment Disorder.** The defiance is in reaction to a life stressor, such as divorce, excessive school expectations, or birth of a sibling.
- **Conduct Disorder.** The misbehavior is more severe and pervasive.
- **ADHD.** The child also has hyperactivity, impulsivity, and/or inattentiveness.
- **Bipolar or Depressive Disorders.** The irritability arises from clear depressive or manic symptoms.
- **Separation Anxiety Disorder.** The opposition is focused on resisting separations.

Diagnostic Tips

- **Caution in using the diagnosis.** Children almost always disappoint their parents at some time or other. ODD should not be diagnosed casually whenever a child is not getting along well with one or both parents. It should persist and occur across different environments.
- **Role of family expectations.** The child's "defiance" may be an expectable reaction to parental perfectionism and excessive demands.
- **Relation to Conduct Disorder.** ODD may in some kids be a milder form of, or prodromal to, Conduct Disorder. But many children with ODD never go on to develop Conduct Disorder, and ODD is an even smaller risk factor for adult Antisocial Personality Disorder.
- **Drugs and defiance.** Always ask about substance use in teenagers because it is the most common source of parent–child confrontation.
- **Giving priority to other disorders.** ODD is usually not a meaningful add-on if the authority struggles are a complication of ADHD, a Bipolar or Depressive Disorder, or an Anxiety Disorder.

312.9 Unspecified Disruptive Behavior Disorder

Don't use Unspecified Disruptive Behavior Disorder as a "back door" for Disruptive Mood Dysregulation Disorder, which is likely to be overdiagnosed in children with normal temper tantrums (see the Caution box at the end of Chapter 3 about the latter diagnosis).

■ 299.00 AUTISM SPECTRUM DISORDER

Screening Question

"Does your child avoid interpersonal contact, not understand social cues, repeat strange stereotyped behaviors, or have language problems?"

Diagnostic Prototype

DSM-5 has collapsed into one large Autism Spectrum Disorder that had previously been separate categories for Autistic Disorder (severe classic autism) and milder Asperger's Disorder, which did not include language impairment. Below are the prototypes for each.

Autistic Disorder (Severe Classic Autism)

Severe classic autism is unmistakable. The problems arise early in infancy and gravely impoverish the child's social interaction, language development, and behavioral repertoire. He lacks an inbuilt and automatic ability to understand and respond to social cues or to enjoy social interaction. The usual eye contact, fond gazing, smiling, hugging, and expression of emotion that enrich our interpersonal lives are absent. Language is slow in coming, extremely limited, peculiar, stereotyped, and noncommunicative. Behaviors are ritualistic, inflexibly repetitive, preoccupying, and not goal-directed.

Asperger's Disorder

Asperger's Disorder is a milder form of autism that does not require the presence of language impairment. It was added as a separate diagnosis by DSM-IV, but has been dropped as a term in DSM-5. Instead, what previously was called Asperger's is included as part of the DSM-5 Autism Spectrum.

The Wider Autism Spectrum

Autism Spectrum Disorder includes the two prototypes above, but also describes a heterogeneous group of people who no longer embody any one clear prototype. Problems include peculiar nonverbal communication; eccentricity in interests and manner; ritualized, repetitive, restricted behaviors; strong sensory sensitivities and inflexible preferences; lack of interpersonal intimacy, reciprocity, and pleasure; and severe social awkwardness/isolation. These occur in varying combinations and severities that make diagnosis difficult. This loose usage accounts in part for the recent 20-fold increase in the rate of diagnosis of Autism.

Differential Diagnosis:
Rule These Conditions Out

- **Neurological illnesses with onset in infancy or early childhood.** One such illness is Rett's Disorder, which was included in DSM-IV, but has been dropped from DSM-5.
- **Intellectual Developmental Disorder.** The child has a low IQ score without characteristic social disconnectedness and ritualistic behaviors.
- **Learning Disorder.** There are specific academic deficits without the characteristic autistic behaviors.
- **OCD.** The child may have strange rituals, but OCD usually has a later onset, normal attachment, and intact language.
- **Social Anxiety Disorder (Social Phobia).** There is social awkwardness, but not the other social, speech, and behavioral idiosyncrasies.
- **Schizophrenia.** There is a later onset, and delusions or hallucinations are present.
- **Schizotypal Personality Disorder.** This usually has a later onset, but there is considerable overlap.
- **Normal eccentricity.** The behaviors reflect individual differences and don't cause clinically significant distress or impairment.

Diagnostic Tips

- **Exploding rates.** Autism Spectrum Disorder used to be extremely rare but has increased 20-fold in recent years, so that it is now diagnosed in more than 1% of the general population.

- **Reasons for the epidemic.** These rapid changes in rates are due to relabeling, not to an actual change in the rate of autistic behaviors. Some of the increase in prevalence is due to increased awareness, reduced stigma, and the diagnosis of much milder cases. Much of it is due to loose diagnosis/inaccurate labeling because a diagnosis of Autism Spectrum Disorder is a prerequisite for extra school services. Mild autism is very hard to distinguish from normal eccentricity and social awkwardness, and from other causes of disturbed behavior and learning problems. With so much on the line, clinicians often feel pressured in doubtful boundary cases into making an Autism Spectrum Disorder diagnosis.

- **Avoiding overdiagnosis.** The Autism Spectrum does not have clear boundaries with normal eccentricity, Social Anxiety Disorder (Social Phobia), OCD and related disorders, Schizotypal Personality Disorder, Intellectual Developmental Disorder, and neurological problems. The symptoms must be severe and persistent, must cause clinically significant impairment, and must not be better explained by another condition.

- **Stability of diagnosis.** Autism Spectrum Disorder is meant to describe persistent and pervasive problems, but because of loose diagnosis, half the kids now thus labeled autistic are quickly "outgrowing" it.

- **Stigma.** Although the stigma of the Autism Spectrum is greatly reduced, it certainly hasn't disappeared. Those who have been mislabeled often feel scarred.

- **Reduced expectations.** Mislabeling people as having Autism Spectrum Disorder may reduce what they feel they can accomplish and close doors that would otherwise have been open to them.

- **Preserving individual differences.** Eccentricity is the spice of life, not necessarily a symptom of psychiatric illness. Severe classic autism is perhaps the most impairing of all the mental disorders, but the milder forms of Autism Spectrum Disorder merge imperceptibly into normal individual difference that we should embrace, not pathologize.

- **Decoupling from services.** Many kids desperately need special educational programs that currently are available only if they receive a diagnosis of Autism Spectrum Disorder. It would be better for them and would lead to more accurate diagnosis if eligibility for the needed school services was based more on an individualized evaluation of their real educational needs, and less on what has become a vague, broadly inclusive, and not very predictive definition of Autism. The services are surely needed, but a DSM diagnosis is not necessarily a useful or specific way of assigning them.

- **Risk–benefit ratio.** The loose diagnosis of Autism Spectrum Disorder solves some problems, but creates its own set of risks for those who are mislabeled.

■ 309.21 SEPARATION ANXIETY DISORDER

Screening Question

"Is your child inordinately scared of separations?"

Diagnostic Prototype

The child goes ballistic when left behind and is terrified of being alone. The worries about having to go to school tomorrow begin almost as soon as the child gets home from school today. Clinging to a parent, she complains of a stomachache, diarrhea, or a headache and begins persistent begging and bargaining for even one day off. As bedtime approaches, the child finds endless excuses to stay up and refuses to let the parent leave the bedroom until she falls asleep. The child is afraid of bad dreams, is frequently wakened by them, and winds up spending the night sleeping in the parents' bed. When morning comes, she frets, whines, kicks, screams, and does a sit-in before finally being forced onto the school bus. The child has no friends because she won't leave home for play dates, and peers call her "baby" and "scaredy-cat."

Differential Diagnosis: Rule These Conditions Out

- **Normal developmental anxiety.** Separation anxiety that is transient and doesn't cause impairment.
- **Adjustment Disorder.** Anxiety that is an expectable reaction to stress

(e.g., divorce, parental hospitalization) but causes clinically significant distress or impairment.

- **Another mental disorder.** Separation problems that are part of a more general clinical presentation (e.g., a Depressive Disorder, Generalized Anxiety Disorder, Panic Disorder, Autism Spectrum Disorder).

Diagnostic Tips

- **Evolution.** Separation fears have huge survival value: Kids who didn't complain over separations were left behind or eaten by tigers. Our ancestors were the "scaredy-cats" who kept their parents close; that is why separation fears are so common and normal.
- **Developmental factors.** There is a wide range of normal fears, and the diagnosis should be made only when the fears are not age-appropriate and there is significant impairment.
- **Cultural factors.** Norms regarding the relative value of independence versus dependence vary greatly across cultures. Separation fears should considerably exceed what is expectable in a given culture.
- **Stress.** Transient separation problems occurring after stress do not constitute a mental disorder.
- **Diagnosis in adults.** Separation Anxiety Disorder is usually a disorder of childhood, but may rarely be diagnosed in adults if onset is before age 18 and if separation fears aren't better explained as part of another disorder.
- **Course.** Most kids eventually grow out of their excessive fear of separation, but for a few it is a prelude to an adult Anxiety Disorder.

■ 319 INTELLECTUAL DEVELOPMENTAL DISORDER

Screening Question

"Is your child a slow learner?" "Is this causing problems?"

Diagnostic Prototype

An IQ test reveals a low score (the DSM-IV cutoff was 70), and the individual also has low scores on tests of adaptive functioning.

Differential Diagnosis: Rule These Conditions Out

- **Borderline Intellectual Functioning.** The IQ is above 70. Code this V62.89.

- **Autism Spectrum Disorder.** There are also serious defects in social interaction and stereotypic behaviors.

- **Learning Disorder.** The problem is specific to learning, rather than generalized to all intellectual functions.

- **Major Neurocognitive Disorder (Dementia).** Onset is after age 18.

- **Malingering.** The person seeks to avoid legal or other responsibility by feigning intellectual incapacity.

- **Other mental disorders.** Depressive Disorders, Anxiety Disorders, and others may interfere with intellectual functioning.

Diagnostic Tips

- **IQ testing.** Intellectual Developmental Disorder is not a diagnosis that can be based only on a clinical interview. It requires individualized IQ testing and individualized testing of adaptive functioning, each done by someone expert in the respective fields and familiar with the child's language and cultural background.

- **Error of measurement.** There is measurement error inherent in any testing procedure. Again, the DSM-IV cutoff IQ score for Intellectual Developmental Disorder was 70, but this has to be interpreted within the context of the entire clinical situation.

- **IQ scores above 70.** Slightly higher IQ scores (plus 5 points) may be consistent with the diagnosis of Intellectual Developmental Disorder if there are also clear problems in adaptive functioning.

- **Misleadingly low IQ scores.** IQ scores below 70 can be compatible with no diagnosis if there are no problems in adaptive functioning and/or if the person was uncooperative, inattentive, anxious, depressed, sleep-deprived, or suffering from another mental disorder during the time of testing.

- **Other reasons for low scores.** IQ scores may not be particularly informative if someone is not fluent in the language of the test, has been educationally deprived, is culturally unfamiliar with the content being tested, has severe learning disabilities, or is malingering.

- **Test consistency.** The pattern of test scores is more important than the score on any given test. The scores on repeated tests should cluster around a true score. When there is marked variability, the higher scores are likely to be the more indicative, since there are many reasons why a given score might underestimate a person's intelligence, but no reason why scores should overestimate it.

- **Age of onset.** This must be before age 18. Similar intellectual problems occurring with an onset after 18 would be classified as Major Neurocognitive Disorder (Dementia).

- **Severity.** Most people with the diagnosis of Intellectual Developmental Disorder would be classified as having it in the range of mild severity, and usually don't have a clearly defined etiology. The more severe the problem, the more likely it is that a specific cause can be found on thorough workup.

- **Comorbid mental disorders.** These often present atypically and are difficult to diagnose accurately in the presence of Intellectual Developmental Disorder. Evaluation is also limited because the person may not be a particularly good informant. Using an Unspecified diagnosis as described in Chapter 1 is preferable to making a more specific diagnosis based on unsupportable inferences. For example, Unspecified Psychotic Disorder may be more accurate than a diagnosis of Schizophrenia in someone with Intellectual Developmental Disorder who develops hallucinations or delusions.

- **Relation to Autism.** Intellectual Developmental Disorder and Autism Spectrum Disorder can both be diagnosed when both are present.

- **Learning Disorder.** These can also be diagnosed if the learning problem is disproportionate to what would be expected from the person's IQ.

■ LEARNING DISORDER

Specify if:

315.00 **Reading (special problems in reading comprehension, speed, or accuracy)**

315.1 **Mathematics (special problems in arithmetic, copying numbers or signs, or recognizing them)**

314.2 **Written Expression (special problems with grammar, sentence structure, or organization)**

315.9 **Unspecified**

Screening Question

"Does your child have a problem with reading, writing, or math?"

Diagnostic Prototype

Performance on the specific area of academic testing is very far below what might be expected given the person's age and overall IQ, as well as the quality of previous education. The impairments interfere with school, work, or other aspects of life functioning.

Differential Diagnosis: Rule These Conditions Out

- **Intellectual Developmental Disorder.** The specific learning problems are no greater than what would be expected from the person's overall IQ score.
- **Autism Spectrum Disorder.** This is the cause of poor functioning, but both diagnoses can be given together if a specific academic area is disproportionately impaired.
- **Sensory deficit.** This accounts for the learning problems.
- **ADHD.** It causes poor test taking, but both diagnoses can be given together whenever appropriate.

Diagnostic Tips

- **Need for an expert diagnostician.** Most mental health clinicians do not have the testing skills or specialized knowledge to diagnose Learning Disorder. Referral to an expert or reliance on test results reported in previous records will almost always be necessary.
- **Individualized testing.** This is necessary to ensure that the learning difficulties are not caused by cultural or language barriers, lack of cooperation, or the presence of another disorder (e.g., ADHD).
- **Combined problems.** A person with one type of Learning Disorder often has more than one. Code all that apply.
- **Age of discovery.** Learning Disorder is usually picked up in the lower grades in kids who have average or low IQs. Brighter children may not be identified as having the disorder until they enter higher grades, when the work becomes more difficult.

■ FEEDING DISORDERS

307.52 Pica

Screening Question

"Does your child eat strange things like paint or dirt?"

Diagnostic Prototype

The child persistently eats stuff that has no food value.

Differential Diagnosis:
Rule These Conditions Out

- **Normal behavior.** The behavior is normal in toddlers up to about 2 years old.
- **Culturally accepted ritual.**
- **Psychotic Disorders.** The person eats strange stuff in response to a hallucination or delusion.
- **Nutritional deficiency or starvation.**

Diagnostic Tips

- **Developmental stage.** Don't diagnose Pica in toddlers. The disorder can occur in older kids with low IQ.
- **Frequency.** The behavior must happen often enough to be a problem.
- **Preferences.** Dirt and paint are the two most common things that are inappropriately ingested.
- **Nutritional compensation.** Some people with iron deficiency anemia develop a craving for iron-rich dirt.

307.53 Rumination Disorder

Screening Question

"Does your child have trouble swallowing food in the usual way?"

Diagnostic Prototype

The child persistently fails to simply swallow food, but instead regurgitates it, chews it again, and then spits it out or swallows it again.

Differential Diagnosis: Rule These Conditions Out

- A gastrointestinal problem.
- Intellectual Developmental Disorder.

Diagnostic Tips

- **Developmental issues.** Rumination Disorder usually occurs in infants or in older children with low IQs.
- **Risks.** Check for malnutrition, weight loss, or failure to thrive.

■ ELIMINATION DISORDERS

787.6 Encopresis With Constipation and Overflow Incontinence

307.7 Encopresis Without Constipation and Overflow Incontinence

Screening Question

"Does your child have toilet-training problems?"

Diagnostic Prototype

A child considered old enough to be toilet-trained defecates repeatedly into underwear or someplace other than a toilet.

Differential Diagnosis: Rule These Conditions Out

- **Normal individual variation.** There is a fairly wide variation in ages at which toilet training is completed.
- **Intellectual Developmental Disorder or Autism Spectrum Disorder.** These may cause delays in toilet training.

Diagnostic Tips

- **Mental age.** The diagnosis should probably not be made in children whose mental age is below 4 years.
- **Cultural variation.** Take into account cultural differences in expectations about when toilet training should be completed.

307.6 Enuresis

Screening Question

"Does your child have toilet-training or bedwetting problems?"

Diagnostic Prototype

A child considered old enough to be toilet-trained urinates repeatedly in bed at night or into underwear during the day. Occasional accidents don't count. The bedwetting should be frequent and persistent over months.

Differential Diagnosis: Rule These Conditions Out

- **Normal individual variation.** There is a fairly wide variation in ages at which toilet training is completed.
- **Intellectual Developmental Disorder or Autism Spectrum Disorder.** These may cause delays in toilet training.

Diagnostic Tips

- **Mental age.** A mental age of about 5 years is the minimum before the Enuresis diagnosis may be appropriate.
- **Cultural variation.** Take into account cultural differences in expectations about when toilet training should be completed.

See Chapter 3 for Caution: Disruptive Mood Dysregulation Disorder.

See Chapter 4 for Caution: The Fad of Childhood Bipolar Disorders.

See Chapter 6 for Tic Disorders.

CHAPTER 3
■ Depressive Disorders

IN THIS CHAPTER:

- Major Depressive Disorder
- CAUTION: Grief versus Major Depressive Disorder
- Chronic Depressive Disorder (Dysthymic Disorder)
- Premenstrual Dysphoric Disorder
- Substance-Induced Depressive Disorder
- Depressive Disorder Due to Another Medical Condition (Indicate the Medical Condition)
- Unspecified Depressive Disorder
- Unspecified Mood Disorder
- CAUTION: Disruptive Mood Dysregulation Disorder

■ MAJOR DEPRESSIVE DISORDER

If Single Episode:

296.21 Major Depressive Disorder, Single Episode, Mild

296.22 Major Depressive Disorder, Single Episode, Moderate

296.23 Major Depressive Disorder, Single Episode, Severe Without Psychotic Features

296.24 Major Depressive Disorder, Single Episode, Severe With Psychotic Features

If Recurrent:

296.31 Major Depressive Disorder, Recurrent, Mild

296.32 Major Depressive Disorder, Recurrent, Moderate

296.33 Major Depressive Disorder, Recurrent, Severe Without Psychotic Features

296.34 Major Depressive Disorder, Recurrent, Severe With Psychotic Features

Screening Question

"Do you ever get so depressed that you can't function?"

Diagnostic Prototype

Shakespeare on depression, in the words of Hamlet: "How weary, stale, flat and unprofitable, seem to me all the uses of this world!" The person feels so deeply down in the dumps and apathetic that she can find no compelling reason to make the laborious climb out of bed. Lacking energy or resolve, she may lie listless and motionless throughout the day. But sometimes depression takes a stormier form, with agitation, restless pacing, irritable snapping, and raging at the fates and at close relatives (think of King Lear on the heath).

The person loses the ability to think clearly, to concentrate, and to make even the simplest decisions. Life seems cardboard and tasteless, drained of pleasure, interest, and excitement. He eats and sleeps too little or too much. Thoughts are slow, heavy, and black, dominated by profound hopelessness, worthlessness, and the weight of unremitting guilt. The only wish is that this "mortal coil" could come to a speedy and decisive end, lifting the constant cloud above and relieving the heavy weight upon the soul.

Heterogeneity

Major Depressive Disorder wears many faces, so expect very varied presentations.

Mood-Congruent Psychotic Features

Depressive preoccupations can become delusional convictions. Some common ones include patients' believing that they are responsible for the death of a loved one or some other catastrophe that was obviously outside their control; being sure that all their money is gone, even when they are presented with healthy financial statements; feeling persecuted by avengers who seem intent on punishing them for unforgivable sins; unshakably believing that they will receive a long jail sentence because of a tax form that was filed a few days late; being certain that they have a cancer or an irreparably damaged or decayed body organ; and so on. Auditory hallucinations may also occur, usually harshly condemning voices vigilantly and viciously attacking the patients for their current thoughts and for their past imagined crimes and misdemeanors.

Mood-Incongruent Psychotic Features

A patient has delusions and hallucinations that are not related to depressive themes and instead are fully equivalent to those that occur in Schizophrenia, but occur only during the depressive episode.

Melancholia

Melancholia is the most severe nonpsychotic form of depression. Nothing can shake the person out of feeling completely terrible. Previous pleasures now hold no interest, and even the best news falls completely flat. The worst hours are upon awakening in the morning because the patient has lost the gift of sleep and wakes up early (often well before dawn) with a churning inability to get back to sleep. The person is without appetite and has to be cajoled or forced to maintain even minimal hydration and nutrition. Some with melancholia are agitated; others are immobile; and still others have alternating features of both.

Reactive Depression

Reactive depression is triggered by external stressors, is less severe and pervasive, and is more responsive to context (e.g., the patient got depressed when she lost her job, but cheers up when people visit, and gets better soon after another job comes through). This is very difficult to distinguish from normal reactions to stress and loss.

Seasonal Pattern

The depression is regularly related to a specific season, usually winter.

Differential Diagnosis: Rule These Conditions Out

- **Bipolar Disorders.** There are current or previous symptoms of Mania or Hypomania (e.g., euphoric mood, grandiosity, not needing sleep, increased productivity and sociability, racing thoughts, impulsivity, spending sprees, reckless sexual behavior).
- **Uncomplicated Bereavement.** The depressive symptoms are better understood as an expectable manifestation of normal grief.
- **Depressive Disorder Due to Another Medical Condition.** Consider this particularly in older patients.
- **Substance-Induced Mood Disorder.** Symptoms are caused by drug abuse, particularly in younger patients, or by medications, particularly in older patients.
- **Chronic Depressive Disorder (Dysthymic Disorder).** Depressive symptoms are milder and persist for years.
- **Schizophrenia, Schizoaffective Disorder, or Delusional Disorder.** Delusions and hallucinations occur during periods when there are no mood symptoms.
- **Brief Psychotic Disorder.** Symptoms occur without a clear episode of depression, resolve quickly, and sometimes arise in response to stress.

Diagnostic Tips

- **Distinguishing Major Depression from normal lows.** At the mild end of the severity spectrum, Major Depressive Disorder must be distinguished from the normal aches, pains, and sufferings of everyday life. The depression must be "dense" (i.e., present for most of the day, almost every day); must last at least a few weeks; and must be severe enough to cause clinically significant impairment.
- **Relation to stressors.** If the symptoms are mild (and especially if they

occur following a job loss, a divorce, or another severe life problem), consider whether what appears to be a Major Depressive Episode is not better understood as a temporary stress reaction. Give it more time to sort itself out before making any definitive diagnosis. The DSM's 2-week duration requirement for a Major Depressive Episode is a general compromise that covers most situations reasonably well, but does not always make sense for a given patient. Don't jump to the diagnosis in mild and reactive cases. Whenever you are in doubt, watchfully wait for 4 weeks (or even longer) to see how things develop.

- **Diagnosis in the young.** Be cautious about making the diagnosis of Major Depressive Disorder in children and teenagers. First, carefully consider all other factors likely to cause depressive symptoms in kids— especially substance use and family stressors.

- **Diagnosis in the old.** Any late first onset points first to medical illness or medication side effects. Depression in the elderly sometimes causes what appears to be a dementing illness, which clears up when the depression gets better.

- **Engaging the patient.** One-third of severely depressed people don't receive any treatment. Most who finally do see a clinician will have been depressed for months or even years. *Do everything possible to ensure the patient's return for a second visit.* Psychoeducation about the diagnosis of depression and its treatment is a great way to start.

- **Psychotic Major Depression versus Schizoaffective Disorder.** These two near-neighbors are a lot easier to distinguish on paper than in real life. Heated diagnostic arguments about which diagnosis is correct are a complete waste of time and brainpower. Patients at this boundary defy any precise sorting to one or the other side of it. They should be seen as and treated for what they are—patients at the boundary. Unspecified Psychotic Disorder should end the discussion.

- **Course.** This can be very variable. Some episodes of Major Depressive Disorder last for weeks; most last many months; less frequently, some last years; some last a lifetime. People can have just a single episode or more than 20. After a first episode, there is a 50% chance of having another. The second episode raises to 70% the chance of a third. After four episodes, expect that more will come in the future. For any given episode, about one in three patients gets completely well; one in three gets much better but still has some remaining symptoms; one in three doesn't respond at all to the first treatment and needs to try another.

CAUTION:
Grief versus Major Depressive Disorder

The symptoms of grief (sadness, loss of interest, reduced energy, difficulty sleeping and eating) are completely equivalent to the symptoms of mild Major Depression. Previous DSMs have recognized this by having an explicit "Bereavement exclusion," suggesting that Major Depressive Disorder not be diagnosed in the months following the loss of a loved one unless it presents with severely impairing symptoms such as suicidal ideation, delusions, psychomotor agitation or retardation, or inability to function. DSM-5 has made the serious error of removing this exclusion.

To reduce the harm done by the removal of the Bereavement exclusion, DSM-5 includes a note that attempts to distinguish the symptoms of grief from those of Major Depressive Disorder and encourages clinical judgment in reducing diagnostic exuberance. Take advantage of this note to avoid the overdiagnosis and overtreatment of Major Depressive Disorder in individuals who are experiencing normal, expectable, and necessary grief. Reserve the diagnosis only for those who have had previous Major Depressive Episodes and/or are now having severe and prolonged symptoms. In a similar way, other life stressors like job loss, divorce, or financial problems can cause symptoms that are equivalent to those of mild Major Depression, but are completely understandable in the context within which they occur. I again recommend avoiding excessive diagnosis and treatment whenever symptoms are proportional to the loss or stress.

■ 300.4 CHRONIC DEPRESSIVE DISORDER (DYSTHYMIC DISORDER)

Screening Question

"Are you almost always depressed?"

Diagnostic Prototype

The depression is a mild but almost constant presence. There are some good days and some especially bad days, but most days are dull gray. Symptoms of depression (hopelessness, poor self-image, guilt, worthlessness; social withdrawal; problems with appetite, sleep, energy) are present, but in a much less severe register than in Major Depressive Disorder. The person is able to function and to keep the depression fairly well hidden, except to those who know her well. But life is an ongoing and unremitting burden.

Differential Diagnosis: Rule These Conditions Out

- **Normal existential sadness.** Persistent sadness can be normal, especially in people who must cope with chronically stressful or disappointing lives.
- **Chronic Major Depressive Disorder.** The symptoms are severe.
- **Bipolar Disorders.** There have been Manic or Hypomanic Episodes.
- **Depressive Disorder Due to Another Medical Condition.** The physiological aspects of an illness (e.g., anemia or hypothyroidism) cause long-term depressive symptoms.
- **Substance-Induced Depressive Disorder.** There is substance use that is also chronic.
- **Chronic Psychotic Disorders.** Chronic depression is an associated feature, but it is not diagnosed separately.

Diagnostic Tips

- **Informants.** It is in the nature of things that people retrospectively distort the past, based on their feeling states in the present. People who are depressed now may naturally exaggerate the duration and severity of their lifetime depression. Having informants is useful.
- **Boundary with normal sadness.** Lots of people are chronically sad and pessimistic. The diagnosis of Chronic Depressive Disorder should be reserved only for those who have clinically significant distress or impairment.
- **Boundary with Major Depressive Disorder.** Major Depression takes priority over Chronic Depressive Disorder if the depressive symptoms are a continuation of a Major Depressive Episode.
- **Relation to a chronic stressor.** It doesn't make sense to diagnose a mental disorder if the person's level of sadness is proportional to long-standing and very difficult life circumstances, like unemployment, chronic financial pressure, having to care for a spouse with dementia, or coping with having a chronic illness.
- **Relation to Personality Disorder.** When Chronic Depressive Disorder and a Personality Disorder coexist (and they often do), it may be useful to diagnose both.

- **Relation to Bipolar Disorders.** Chronic Depressive Disorder is by definition unipolar and not compatible with a Manic or Hypomanic Episode.
- **Relation to medical illness.** Be especially suspicious of a medical illness if onset is late in life.
- **Relation to chronic substance use.** When substance use is involved, the only way to tease out cause from effect is to get the person off the substance(s)—which is admittedly not easy to do.

■ 625.4 PREMENSTRUAL DYSPHORIC DISORDER

Screening Question

"Do you have lots of psychological and physical symptoms occurring around the time of your menstrual periods?"

Diagnostic Prototype

The patient's menstrual periods are consistently preceded by depression, irritability, suddenly changeable or reactive mood, and anxiety. She may also experience reduced energy and interest, changes in sleep or appetite, and trouble concentrating or getting things done, as well as a variety of physical symptoms.

Differential Diagnosis:
Rule These Conditions Out

- **Normal premenstrual discomfort.** Symptoms are mild, are transient, and occur only during some cycles.
- **Premenstrual exacerbation of another mental disorder.** The symptoms persist throughout the menstrual cycle, but get worse around the time of menses.
- **Premenstrual exacerbation of dysphoria caused by a general medical condition.** Examples of such conditions include hypothyroidism, systemic lupus, anemia, and cancer.

Diagnostic Tips

- **Severity.** Premenstrual discomfort is very common and should not be considered a mental disorder. The diagnosis of Premenstrual Dysphoric Disorder should be used only when there are prominent psychological (not just physical) symptoms and when these cause significant distress or impairment.
- **Persistence.** The diagnosis should be made only when the dysphoria occurs with most periods for at least a year.
- **Oral contraceptives.** The diagnosis is not to be made if the symptoms occur only during contraceptive use.
- **Prospective daily ratings.** These should be done for several cycles to confirm that symptoms are closely related to the menses. Retrospective reporting is often misleading.

■ SUBSTANCE-INDUCED DEPRESSIVE DISORDER

291.89 If Alcohol-Induced
292.84 If Induced by Any Other Substance (Indicate Substance)

Screening Question

"Might your depressions be related to your use of alcohol, drugs, or medications?"

Diagnostic Prototype

The depressive symptoms are caused by a substance taken recreationally, a prescribed medication, or exposure to a toxin.

Differential Diagnosis: Rule These Conditions Out

- **A primary Depressive Disorder.** The substance use is incidental, unrelated, or secondary to the depression.
- **Substance Intoxication or Withdrawal.** The depressive symptoms are

no greater in severity or longer in duration than would be expected in simple Substance Intoxication or Withdrawal.

- **Depression Due to Another Medical Condition.** An example of such a condition is hypothyroidism.

Diagnostic Tips

- **Chronology.** The substance use should begin or increase before the onset of the depressive symptoms. Withdrawing the substance should, within a month or so, result in the disappearance or significant reduction of the depressive symptoms.
- **Severity.** A primary Depressive Disorder is more likely if symptoms are much more severe than expected, given the type and amount of the substance used.
- **Age-related factors.** In younger people, be sure to take a careful history of substance use before assuming that the depression is primary. In older people, depression is more likely to be a side effect of prescribed medication, especially if they are taking a number of medications that may be interacting with one another.
- **Laboratory testing.** People are sometimes not "up front" about disclosing substance use. Testing for alcohol, recreational drug, and medication use is probably underutilized as a diagnostic tool. *I strongly recommend it.*

■ 293.83 DEPRESSIVE DISORDER DUE TO ANOTHER MEDICAL CONDITION (INDICATE THE MEDICAL CONDITION)

Screening Question

"Please tell me about your medical illnesses and their treatment."

Diagnostic Prototype

The depressive symptoms are caused by the direct physiological effects of a medical condition.

Differential Diagnosis: Rule These Conditions Out

- **A primary Depressive Disorder.** The medical illness is incidental, unrelated, or secondary to the depression.
- **Adjustment Disorder.** Depressive symptoms are a psychological response to the illness, not due to its physiological effects.
- **Substance-Induced Depressive Disorder.** Symptoms may be a side effect of the medication used for treating the medical illness.

Diagnostic Tips

- **Chronology.** The medical illness should begin before the onset of the depressive symptoms, and improvements in the medical illness should result in the disappearance or significant reduction of the depressive symptoms.
- **Severity.** A primary Depressive Disorder is more likely if symptoms are much more severe than expected, given the type and severity of the medical illness.
- **Age-related factors.** There should be a high index of suspicion that medical illness may be involved if someone develops a first onset of depression after age 50.
- **Medical examination and laboratory testing.** A thorough medical examination is indicated to pin down the diagnosis of the medical illness.
- **Mechanism.** This diagnosis applies only when the depression is caused by the *direct physiological effects of the medical illness on brain functioning*. It is not to be used when the depression is a psychological reaction to being sick. Depending on the severity and duration, depression due to a psychological reaction to illness should not be diagnosed at all (if it is not clinically significant); should be diagnosed as Adjustment Disorder (subthreshold to Major Depressive Disorder, but with clinical significance); or should be diagnosed as Major Depressive Disorder.
- **Interaction with medication side effects.** It can be very difficult to tease out whether it is the illness or the medication that is causing depression. Often it may be both.

■ 311 UNSPECIFIED DEPRESSIVE DISORDER

Use the diagnosis of Unspecified Depressive Disorder when you have determined that there is a depressive disorder, but there is not enough information to distinguish which one best fits. Often it takes the passage of time and several visits to determine the possible impact of substances or medical illness. This category would also be used for presentations of depression that don't resemble any of the specific categories described above but still cause clinically significant distress or impairment.

■ 296.90 UNSPECIFIED MOOD DISORDER

DSM-5 has made the mistake of dropping what was Mood Disorder Not Otherwise Specified in DSM-IV. This creates a hole in its classification for the fairly common situation of a patient who clearly has a Mood Disorder, but one that has not yet clearly declared itself as unipolar or bipolar. I recommend that you feel comfortable using Unspecified Mood Disorder (use the ICD-9-CM code for Mood Disorder Not Elsewhere Classified) when you have determined that there is a Mood Disorder, but there is not enough information to distinguish it as a Depressive Disorder or a Bipolar Disorder. Time and further evaluation will tell.

CAUTION:
Disruptive Mood Dysregulation Disorder

DSM-5 has introduced the Disruptive Mood Dysregulation Disorder (DMDD) diagnosis to describe children who have frequent temper tantrums. Its inclusion is based on minimal research and was justified only by the need to reduce the overdiagnosis of Childhood Bipolar Disorders (see my Caution box on the latter in Chapter 4). I fear that DMDD will cause more harm than good, and I strongly recommend that it be used extremely sparingly, if at all. The problems with DMDD are as follows:

1. It is impossible to distinguish DMDD from temper tantrums occurring in normal children. The result will be false-positive misidentification of normal but annoying kids as mentally disordered.
2. It is impossible to distinguish DMDD from temper tantrums occurring in other

psychiatric disorders. DMDD may therefore distract attention away from the appropriate differential diagnosis of irritability in children.

3. As with Childhood Bipolar Disorders, there may be an effort by drug companies to promote use of harmful medications, particularly antipsychotics that can cause large weight gains (and thus the risk of obesity, diabetes, and heart disease).

For safety's sake, I recommend that a careful stepped procedure be followed in diagnosing irritable children with frequent temper tantrums (see Chapter 1). DMDD should either not be used at all or should be used with great caution and under special circumstances, and it should certainly not be regarded as an indication for medication use except in extreme situations. In my view, DMDD is not ready for prime time.

CHAPTER 4
■ Bipolar Disorders

IN THIS CHAPTER:

- Bipolar I Disorder
- CAUTION: The Fad of Childhood Bipolar Disorders
- Bipolar II Disorder
- Cyclothymic Disorder
- Substance-Induced Bipolar Disorder
- Bipolar Disorder Due to Another Medical Condition (Indicate the Medical Condition)
- Unspecified Bipolar Disorder
- Unspecified Mood Disorder

■ 296.XX BIPOLAR I DISORDER

Fourth-Digit Codes:

.0x Bipolar I Disorder, Single Manic Episode

.40 Bipolar I Disorder, Most Recent Episode Hypomanic

.4x Bipolar I Disorder, Most Recent Episode Manic

.5x Bipolar I Disorder, Most Recent Episode Depressed

.6x Bipolar I Disorder, Most Recent Episode Mixed

.7 Bipolar I Disorder, Most Recent Episode Unspecified

Fifth-Digit Codes:

.x1 Mild

.x2 Moderate

.x3 Severe

.x4 Severe With Psychotic Features

.x5 In Partial Remission

.x6 In Full Remission

.x0 Unspecified

Screening Question

"Do you have mood swings—sometimes way up, other times way down?"

Diagnostic Prototype

The ups in Bipolar I Disorder can be wonderful—at least for a while. The world is the patient's oyster. Everything feels so smooth, so easy, so great, and so vivid. Colors are brighter, food is more delicious, sex is more intense, jokes are funnier. The patient is flying high with expansive ideas, vaulting ambitions, booming confidence, and dauntless energy. His mind is racing, his speech is pressured and punning, and his body is in perpetual motion. There is nothing he can't do, and the usual limitations in life no longer apply. There seems no need for sleep or eating, or for the routine drudgery of the everyday. "So much to do and so little time." Impulses are unleashed—wild shopping sprees, reckless investing, expansive new projects, intense new relationships, fast cars, adventurous drugs, restless travel. "Bring it on."

Eventually, the euphoria morphs from high spirits into impatient irritability (especially when other people refuse to join the party). Increased energy merges into restless agitation, then dissolves into utter exhaustion; expansive thoughts can become psychotic delusions. At the end of every Manic Episode, there is an inevitable crash with a bruising collapse into depression. Some people have Mixed Episodes from the very start, with rapidly alternating manic and depressive symptoms, and with lots of irritability, agitation, and insomnia. The first episode of Bipolar I Disorder is usually before age 35, and most people have many lifetime episodes. Some are on a particularly rough roller coaster, with rapid cycling from

mania to depression again and again, with few respites of normal functioning. The Depressive Episodes are equivalent to those in Major Depressive Disorder as described in Chapter 3. Depression predominates in most
patients with Bipolar I.

Differential Diagnosis: Rule These Conditions Out

- **Major Depressive Disorder.** The person with depressive symptoms
  has never had Manic or Hypomanic Episodes.
- **Bipolar II Disorder.** The person has had Hypomanic Episodes, but
  never a full Manic Episode.
- **Cyclothymic Disorder.** Lesser mood swings of alternating depression and hypomania never reach the full register of Major Depressive
  or Manic Episodes, but they still cause clinically significant distress or
  impairment.
- **Normal mood swings.** There are alternating periods of sadness and
  elevated mood, but without clinically significant distress or impairment.
- **Schizoaffective Disorder.** Symptoms resemble Bipolar I Disorder,
  Severe With Psychotic Features, but psychotic symptoms occur even
  when mood symptoms are not present.
- **Schizophrenia or Delusional Disorder.** Psychotic symptoms dominate
  the clinical presentation and occur without prominent mood episodes.
- **Bipolar Disorder Due to Another Medical Condition.** Examples of
  such conditions include stroke and hyperthyroidism.
- **Substance-Induced Bipolar Disorder.** For example, stimulant drugs
  can produce bipolar symptoms.
- **Caution: Disruptive Mood Dysregulation Disorder.** DMDD was
  designed as an alternative to childhood Bipolar Disorders, but I advise
  against using this diagnosis. See my more extensive caution at the end
  of Chapter 3.

Diagnostic Tips

- **Mania as a diagnostic emergency.** Manic patients have terrible judgment and get themselves into all sorts of interpersonal, financial, legal,
  and sexual trouble. The combination of grandiosity, impulsivity, delu-

sions, and heightened energy can lead to fatal car accidents, "flying" off a roof, quick intimacy with dangerous strangers, or lethal drug overdose.

- **Noncompliance.** Unfortunately, manic patients also resent being reined in, are quick to travel to distant places, deny the need for treatment, and barely notice that you exist. The odds that such a patient will show up for a second visit are not great. Assume you have to do something right now.

- **Hospitalization.** Admission to a hospital is often necessary for clearer diagnosis, for beginning the treatment, and (most important) for safety.

- **Informants.** People close to the patient can supply important information and can help keep the patient involved in treatment rather than taking the next plane to anywhere.

- **Unipolar Manic Episodes.** A very small percentage of patients with Bipolar I have had only Manic, never Depressive, Episodes. They are usually men, and most do go on later to have Major Depressive Episodes.

- **Mixed Episodes.** Mixed Episodes count toward a diagnosis of Bipolar I, but can be very difficult to distinguish from unipolar agitated depression. When in doubt, stick to the diagnosis of Major Depression unless there is a family history of Bipolar Disorders.

- **Role of substances.** Medications and other substances sometimes cause Manic Episodes in patients previously diagnosed with Depressive Disorders. Whether their diagnostic status is best considered unipolar or bipolar is controversial. Factors that tip the diagnosis toward Bipolar I include a family history of Bipolar Disorders; previous equivocal Mixed or Hypomanic Episodes; a previous substance-induced mania; and/or disproportionately severe or enduring manic symptoms.

- **Late onset.** Whenever there is a first Manic Episode after age 35, always consider the possible role of a medical illness, an antidepressant medication, or other substances.

- **Schizoaffective Disorder.** As noted above, this is often very difficult to distinguish from Bipolar I Disorder, Severe With Psychotic Features. At the boundary, the distinction is probably without a difference. Go ahead and diagnose Unspecified Psychotic Disorder.

- **Avoiding overdiagnosis of childhood Bipolar Disorders.** Most irritability and temper tantrums in childhood are either normal or associated with ADHD, Conduct Disorder, or ODD, and are not related to Bipolar Disorders. Don't join the fad. (See the Caution box below.)

CAUTION:
The Fad of Childhood Bipolar Disorders

The rate of diagnosis for childhood Bipolar Disorders has increased 40-fold in the last 20 years, with consequent massive overusage of antipsychotic and mood-stabilizing medication. Most kids who now get the diagnosis have nonepisodic temper outbursts and irritability—not classic swings between Manic or Hypomanic Episodes and Depressive Episodes. The idea that Bipolar Disorders present very differently in children is largely untested.

"Leading" researchers, heavily sponsored by drug companies, encouraged child clinicians, educators, and parents to ignore the standard Bipolar Disorder definitions and instead to entertain the diagnosis of childhood Bipolar Disorders in a free-form, overinclusive way.

The "epidemic" of childhood Bipolar Disorders fed off the engaging story line that (1) they are extremely common; (2) they were previously greatly underdiagnosed; (3) they present differently in children because of developmental factors; (4) they can explain the variety of childhood emotional dysregulation; and (5) they have diverse presenting symptoms (e.g., irritability, anger, agitation, aggression, distractibility, hyperactivity, and conduct problems).

Problems with the Diagnosis

The boundaries of childhood Bipolar Disorders have pushed far into unfamiliar territory to label kids who previously received other diagnoses (e.g., ADHD, Conduct Disorder, ODD, or Anxiety Disorders) or no diagnosis at all ("temperamental" but normal kids). The other more specific causes of irritability may be missed. For example, ADHD often presents with an irritability that responds best to stimulants, but these may be withheld in the face of an incorrect Bipolar Disorder diagnosis. Normal development should always be the first thought for irritable teenagers, and Substance Abuse for severely irritable teens.

A Lifetime Diagnosis

The diagnosis of a Bipolar Disorder carries the connotation that it will last a lifetime and require continuous medication treatment. It is unwise to base such a consequential judgment on such a short track record in children and teenagers. Many causes of temper outbursts are much shorter-lived and amenable to time-limited treatment.

Inappropriate and Excessive Medication Use

Teenagers, children, and even infants have been overmedicated with antipsychotics and mood-stabilizing drugs that can promote obesity, diabetes, and heart disease, and possibly reduce lifespan.

Stigma and Risk

The label of a Bipolar Disorder can distort a person's life narrative and cut off hopes of otherwise achievable ambitions. Those labeled worry about getting married and having children, or about taking on stressful ambitions, jobs, or work challenges. It may become more difficult to get insurance. An incorrect diagnosis of a Bipolar Disorder may reduce one's sense of personal responsibility for, and control over, undesirable behavior. People sometimes use the diagnosis as an excuse for interpersonal or legal problems.

I recommend that the diagnosis of childhood Bipolar Disorders should go back to being rarely used, and that the widespread, inappropriate use of antipsychotics for children and teenagers should be curtailed.

■ 296.89 BIPOLAR II DISORDER

Screening Question

"Do you have mood swings—sometimes going up, other times going down?"

Diagnostic Prototype

Three conditions must be met before Bipolar II Disorder can be diagnosed. First, the person must have Major Depressive Episodes that are fully equivalent to those described in Chapter 3 for unipolar Major Depressive Disorder. Second, she must have at least one clear-cut Hypomanic Episode. Third, the person must never have had a full-blown Manic Episode (if she has had one, that would make the diagnosis Bipolar I, not Bipolar II).

The word "hypomanic" is just a fancy way of saying "less than manic." A Hypomanic Episode is indeed less severe than a Manic Episode, but it has the same symptoms of elevated mood, expansive self-confidence, infectious joking, increased energy, intrusive sociability, and less need for sleep and rest. The mood swing has to be a distinct shift upward from the person's usual gear. The unique thing about a Hypomanic Episode is that it does not usually by itself cause clinically significant impairment or distress.

Differential Diagnosis: Rule These Conditions Out

- **Major Depressive Disorder.** There is no history of Hypomanic Episodes.
- **Bipolar I Disorder.** There has been at least one clear-cut Manic Episode.
- **Cyclothymic Disorder.** Mood swings from hypomania to mild depression cause clinically significant distress or impairment, and there is no history of any Major Depressive Episodes.
- **Normal mood swings.** The person alternately feels a bit high and a bit low, but with no clinically significant distress or impairment.
- **Bipolar Disorder Due to Another Medical Condition.** Examples of such conditions include stroke and hyperthyroidism.
- **Substance-Induced Bipolar Disorder.** The Hypomanic Episode was caused by antidepressant medication or cocaine.
- **ADHD.** ADHD has distractibility, hyperactivity, and impulsivity in common with Bipolar II, but ADHD onset is in early childhood, its course is chronic rather than episodic, and it does not include features of elevated mood.

Diagnostic Tips

- **A difficult decision.** Because it sits on the fuzzy boundary between unipolar Major Depressive Disorder and Bipolar I Disorder, Bipolar II is one of the very toughest diagnostic decisions in all of psychiatry. The diagnosis rests on whether or not the patient has ever had a Hypomanic Episode. Hypomania is difficult to distinguish, particularly if there have been only few and brief episodes and if drugs or medication are a part of the clinical presentation. Always be sure to ask about substance use and prescribed medications.
- **Deciding what's normal.** Hypomanic Episodes are also difficult to distinguish from a normal mood, particularly in someone who has been depressed so much that it feels strange when the depression lifts and

mood returns to normal. For this person, being normal is easily confused with being high.

- **Clues from age of onset.** Bipolar II Disorder usually shows itself before age 35. Whenever there is a late onset, always consider the possibility that a medical illness or substance is causing the symptoms.
- **Family history.** When you are in doubt, a family history of Bipolar Disorders is a useful clue that the patient has underlying Bipolar II Disorder.
- **Other clues.** Rapid cycling in a patient with unipolar Major Depressive Disorder may be a hint of masked Bipolar II Disorder. Agitation or irritability in response to antidepressant medication doesn't clinch the diagnosis but should alert you to it.
- **A high-stakes risk–benefit analysis.** In doubtful boundary cases, it is crucial that this difficult diagnosis be made carefully and correctly. Always do an individualized risk–benefit analysis to decide what will be worse: missing Bipolar II Disorder (and treating with antidepressants alone, which may risk promoting a switch to hypomania, agitation, or rapid cycling) or mistakenly diagnosing Bipolar II Disorder (and giving unnecessary mood stabilizers, which can cause dangerous weight gain with the added risks of diabetes and heart disease). It is often a tough call with no obvious right answer.
- **Unipolar Major Depression first.** When in doubt, diagnose unipolar Major Depressive Disorder. Once the diagnosis of Bipolar II is made, the patient is probably committed to a lifetime course of antipsychotics or mood stabilizers. These should be risked only when really necessary. Withhold the diagnosis of Bipolar II Disorder until there are clear, repeated, or enduring Hypomanic Episodes.
- **Joint decision making.** Educate the patient and family about the risks and benefits on both sides of the unipolar–bipolar divide, and include them in decision making.
- **Severity.** Don't assume that Bipolar II is a milder form of Bipolar I. Although there is no frank Manic Episode in Bipolar II, the Depressive Episodes can be absolutely devastating, and suicide risk can be relatively high.
- **Avoiding overdiagnosis of Bipolar II Disorder.** Rates of Bipolar Disorder diagnoses have doubled since Bipolar II became an official diagnosis in DSM-IV. Some of this resulted from better diagnosis of Bipolar Disorders, but there has also been a tendency to overdiagnose Hypomanic Episodes (stimulated in part by aggressive drug company mar-

keting suggesting that Bipolar Disorders are underdiagnosed and that medication for them is underutilized).

■ 301.13 **CYCLOTHYMIC DISORDER**

Screening Question

"Do you have constant mood swings, alternating from high to low?"

Diagnostic Prototype

The person has alternating hypomanic and depressive symptoms that cause clinically significant distress and impairment, but never severe enough to qualify for Bipolar I or Bipolar II Disorder. These are among the most temperamental, mercurial, unpredictable of people. Catch them on an upswing, and you are their best friend. The conversation is light and breezy; the jokes fly; and soon you are planning an exciting vacation next week. Call them next week, and all bets are off. On the downswing, they want to be left alone, have trouble just getting to work, and couldn't dream of summoning the energy to leave town. The sunny possibilities of hypomania evaporate into a black cloud, and the previously overflowing glass is now much less than half full.

Differential Diagnosis: Rule These Conditions Out

- **Normal mood swings.** The person has ups and downs, but with no clinically significant distress or impairment.
- **Major Depressive Disorder.** There has been a Major Depressive Episode, which rules out Cyclothymic Disorder.
- **Bipolar I Disorder.** There has been at least one Manic Episode, which also rules out Cyclothymic Disorder.
- **Bipolar II Disorder.** Again, there has been at least one clear Major Depressive Episode, which rules out Cyclothymia.
- **Bipolar Disorder Due to Another Medical Condition.** For example, the mood swings are caused by stroke or hyperthyroidism.
- **Substance-Induced Bipolar Disorder.** Mood swings are caused, for example, by antidepressant medication or cocaine.

Diagnostic Tips

- **Normal emotional intensity.** Many people (especially creative ones) have an intense emotional life that is just part of who they are, not evidence of a psychiatric disorder.
- **Magnitude of the swings.** Be sure to reserve the Cyclothymic Disorder diagnosis for mood swings that cause significant distress or impairment but aren't severe enough to qualify for a Bipolar I or Bipolar II diagnosis.
- **Substance use.** Many people go up and down on a roller coaster of intoxication and withdrawal, or they alternate between "uppers" and "downers."
- **Late onset.** Whenever there is a late onset, always consider the possibility of a medical illness.

■ SUBSTANCE-INDUCED BIPOLAR DISORDER

291.89 If Alcohol-Induced
292.84 If Induced by Any Other Substance (Indicate Substance)

Screening Question

"Have you had a lot of mood swings associated with using drugs, drinking alcohol or coffee, taking a medication, or withdrawing from drugs or medication?"

Diagnostic Prototype

Alternating highs and lows often occur as a result of taking or withdrawing from a medication or other substance.

Differential Diagnosis: Rule These Conditions Out

- **Bipolar Disorder Due to Another Medical Condition.** The mood swings come from the medical condition.
- **A primary Bipolar Disorder.** The mood swings preceded the substance use or persist for an extended period after it.

Diagnostic Tips

- **A tough diagnosis.** Establishing that a substance is causing the mood swings can be especially challenging because so many patients with Bipolar Disorders use substances to self-medicate. The following temporal factors provide clues.
- **Onset.** The mood swings start *after* the substance use and (ideally) remit shortly after the substance is stopped.
- **Remission.** The mood swings go away if the person stops the substance and completes a reasonable period of withdrawal.

■ 283.83 BIPOLAR DISORDER DUE TO ANOTHER MEDICAL CONDITION (INDICATE THE MEDICAL CONDITION)

Screening Question

"Have you had mood swings in association with a medical condition, like an overactive thyroid?"

Diagnostic Prototype

Prominent mood swings are caused by the direct physical effects of a medical illness.

Differential Diagnosis: Rule These Conditions Out

- **Substance-Induced Bipolar Disorder.** The mood swings are due to the effects of a medication or other substance.
- **A primary Bipolar Disorder.** The mood swings preceded the medical illness or persist for an extended period after it.

Diagnostic Tips

- **Another tough diagnosis.** Establishing that a medical condition is directly causing the mood swings can be challenging. The following factors support a direct causal relationship.

- **Onset.** The mood swings begin simultaneously with, or shortly after, the onset of the medical condition.
- **Linkage.** There is a close relationship between the severity of the mood swings and the severity of the medical condition (e.g., worsening of symptoms with increasingly high thyroid level in hyperthyroidism).
- **Remission.** Symptoms resolve with successful treatment of the medical condition.
- **Typicality.** There is evidence from the clinical literature that the medical condition in question is known to cause bipolar symptoms in some individuals.

■ 296.80 UNSPECIFIED BIPOLAR DISORDER

Use the diagnosis of Unspecified Bipolar Disorder when a Bipolar Disorder is present, but it is impossible to be specific about whether it is Bipolar I, Bipolar II, or Cyclothymia, or whether it is substance-induced or caused by a general medical condition.

■ 296.90 UNSPECIFIED MOOD DISORDER

Use the diagnosis of Unspecified Mood Disorder (Mood Disorder Not Elsewhere Classified in ICD-9-CM) when a Mood Disorder is present, but it is impossible to be more specific on whether it is unipolar or bipolar, or whether it is substance-induced or caused by a general medical condition. See my discussion of this diagnosis at the end of Chapter 3.

CHAPTER 5

■Anxiety Disorders

IN THIS CHAPTER:

- Panic Disorder
- Agoraphobia
- Social Anxiety Disorder (Social Phobia)
- Specific Phobia
- Generalized Anxiety Disorder
- CAUTION: Overdiagnosis of Generalized Anxiety Disorder
- Anxiety Disorder Due to Another Medical Condition (Indicate the Medical Condition)
- Substance-Induced Anxiety Disorder
- Unspecified Anxiety Disorder

■ PANIC DISORDER

300.21 Panic Disorder With Agoraphobia
300.01 Panic Disorder Without Agoraphobia

Screening Question

"Have you ever had a panic attack?"

Diagnostic Prototype

Panic Disorder feels like being in a cage with a tiger, except that there is no tiger. Suddenly, and seemingly for no reason, the person experiences stark terror along with air hunger, racing heart, dizziness, shaking hands, sweating, a weird feeling of pins and needles in fingers and toes, and a clenching of hands and feet. And all this portends that something even more catastrophic is about to happen soon—perhaps fainting or throwing up, having a heart attack, going crazy, or even dying. Sometimes the world feels unreal, and the person has an uncanny sense of not being himself.

The panic attack is brief and ends almost as suddenly as it began. At first the attacks are not predictably connected to environment triggers, but over time the situations where they have previously occurred may become conditioned cues that provoke new attacks (at least some of the time). The person often then begins to avoid these situations, and as they accumulate, Agoraphobia may eventually develop. Places that prevent ready escape or would cause particular embarrassment are the ones most likely to be avoided.

Differential Diagnosis: Rule These Conditions Out

- **Panic due to exposure to real-life dangers.** Such events as war, a car accident, or rape can induce panic symptoms.
- **Normal occasional panics.** These may have no clinical significance.
- **Substance-Induced Anxiety Disorder.** For example, cocaine use or consumption of too much coffee may induce panic symptoms.
- **Anxiety Disorder Due to Another Medical Condition.** Examples of such conditions include hyperthyroidism and pheochromocytoma.
- **Specific Phobia.** This is triggered by a predictable and specific cue (e.g., snakes, heights, injections).
- **Social Anxiety Disorder (Social Phobia).** This is triggered predictably by exposure to social situations.
- **OCD.** For example, a person with OCD may experience contamination panic if exposed to dirt.
- **Posttraumatic Stress Disorder (PTSD) or Acute Stress Disorder.** Panic symptoms may be cued by reminders of the terrible event.
- **Separation Anxiety Disorder.** This is triggered by separation from a caretaker.
- **Psychotic Disorders.** Panic symptoms may occur in response to delusions or hallucinations.

Diagnostic Tips

- **Real danger.** Panic attacks occurring in response to a significant threat (e.g., being held up at gunpoint) are not the least bit pathological and don't count at all toward a diagnosis of a mental disorder.
- **Panic attacks in normal people.** About 10% of people have occasional, isolated panic attacks that have no clinical significance and shouldn't be diagnosed as Panic Disorder.
- **Duration.** Most panic attacks are extremely brief in duration, lasting less than a half hour. Some people do have interepisode anxiety between attacks, but full-blown terror is not something people can sustain for very long.
- **Hyperventilation.** Many of the physical symptoms are caused by anxious overbreathing and the consequent exhalation of too much carbon dioxide. For diagnostic purposes during the first office visit, you can often provoke the physical symptoms of a panic attack by having the patient hyperventilate voluntarily for a couple of minutes. This exercise is useful in demonstrating the trivial cause of the physical symptoms, thus relieving the patient's fears that there is something radically wrong physically. This also confers a sense of mastery and control over symptoms that previously inspired terror and helplessness. Breathing retraining can be done as part of the initial diagnostic interview, too. Patients who get a lot out of the first visit are much more likely to return for a second.
- **Stress.** Panic Disorder is often provoked or exacerbated during times of life stress and psychological conflict. Getting to know the patient is as important as getting to know the symptoms.
- **Secondary impairments.** Panic attacks often provoke reactions that are much worse than the attacks themselves, particularly Agoraphobia, social withdrawal, generalized anxiety symptoms, and demoralization. Timely and effective diagnosis and treatment are crucial.
- **Substance Intoxication and Withdrawal.** Consider intoxication or withdrawal from alcohol or other substances, and withdrawal from medications (particularly antidepressant and antianxiety drugs), as possible causes or precipitants. Giving up caffeine may help.
- **Late onset.** This is rare enough to suggest an evaluation for medical illness.

- **Importance of a good diagnosis in preventing unnecessary medical tests and treatment.** Patients with Panic Disorder make lots of visits to doctors and emergency rooms before someone realizes that hyperventilation is causing the physical symptoms. It is amazing how often Panic Disorder is missed, resulting in unnecessary testing and irrelevant treatment.
- **Prevention of Agoraphobia.** Effective management of Panic Disorder may prevent the evolution of Agoraphobia. Agoraphobia is a lot easier to prevent than to treat.

■ 300.22 AGORAPHOBIA

Screening Question

"Are there many things you're afraid to do and many places you're afraid to go?"

Diagnostic Prototype

Agoraphobia started with a panic attack that came out of the blue while she was riding on a bus, so she stopped taking buses. She then began having more and more unprovoked panic attacks—first every few weeks, then every week, than every few days. Attending Parents' Night at school risked too much embarrassment. She stopped driving because of fears she would freeze while on the highway. Then an attack at the grocery store placed shopping off limits, and soon she was too afraid to go anywhere by herself. She can't abide the thought of ever standing in lines or being in crowds, lest she have an embarrassing panic attack and not be able to escape from the situation or get help. Movies are completely off limits—too dark and crowded. How could she escape if a panic attack caught her trapped in a middle seat? Planes are out of the question. Her world has progressively shrunk to the small safety zone of the house, and even here she is becoming more uncomfortable when she has to be alone.

In Agoraphobia, feared situations are avoided altogether, endured with intense dread, or entered into only with a trusted "phobic companion." Soon avoidance is the central theme of every aspect of life. Those with this disorder are increasingly imprisoned in what becomes an almost solitary confinement. The crisis that precipitates the first office visit often occurs when the phobic partner feels overwhelmed, becomes impatient, and tries to pull away.

Differential Diagnosis: Rule These Conditions Out

- **Social Anxiety Disorder (Social Phobia).** Only specific social situations are avoided.
- **Specific Phobia.** Only a specific object or situation is avoided.
- **PTSD or Acute Stress Disorder.** The person avoids reminders of a traumatic event.
- **Separation Anxiety Disorder.** The fears motivating avoidance concern separation from a parent or caregiver.
- **OCD.** Avoidance is focused on things that trigger compulsive rituals; for example, a compulsive handwasher avoids dirt.
- **Major Depressive Disorder.** Withdrawal is caused by loss of interest, pleasure, and energy rather than by fears.
- **Psychotic Disorders.** The fears motivating avoidance are delusional.
- **Substance Dependence.** Intoxication and lack of motivation make the person housebound.
- **Malingering.** Avoidance is a manipulation used to bind the phobic partner.

Diagnostic Tips

- **Prevention of Agoraphobia.** As noted above, effective management of Panic Disorder may prevent the evolution of Agoraphobia. Again, Agoraphobia is a lot easier to prevent than to treat.
- **Getting the patient to the first meeting.** The patient will probably dread the psychiatric evaluation at least as much as any of the many other feared situations. It will make the person's appearance at the first visit much more likely if you also invite the phobic companion. The major (really the only) goal of the first visit is to reduce fears and show that you can be helpful, thus raising the odds that the patient will be motivated and comfortable enough to come for a second visit.

- **Embarrassment.** Among all the psychiatric problems, Agoraphobia is one of the most embarrassing to patients. Expect that they will typically disguise or minimize the extent of avoidance. Let them know that you have heard much worse stories many times before, and that the symptoms are well understood and very treatable.

- **The phobic partner.** There will usually be someone who confers safety on the otherwise very dangerous zones the patient is avoiding. Most commonly this is a spouse, parent, or child; sometimes it is a friend or relative; sometimes several people share this role. The patient may not be able to go anywhere alone, but may be able to go everywhere if accompanied by a safe person. The phobic partner is probably sitting in your waiting room. Invite the partner in, and make this person an integral part of the evaluation and treatment.

- **The power of psychoeducation.** Patients with Agoraphobia feel particularly helpless, dependent, and out of control. Psychoeducation provides hope of mastery and reduces the sense of being alone and misunderstood. It will also help the phobic companion to put things in perspective.

- **Relation to panic attacks.** Agoraphobia is usually a secondary complication arising as a consequence of repeated panic attacks. Making this connection with the patient is often a breakthrough and the first step in both diagnosis and treatment.

- **Other triggers.** Not everyone requires full-blown panic attacks to fuel the pattern of avoidance. Especially in an elderly patient, fears of becoming dizzy or of falling down in a public place may gradually reduce the patient's safety zone.

- **Social Anxiety Disorder and Specific Phobia.** These sometimes become more severe and generalized, with more and more things avoided, until they evolve gradually into Agoraphobia.

- **Substance use.** Agoraphobia and substance misuse are closely linked. Using substances for self-medication can get out of hand and evolve into Substance Dependence. Anxiolytic medications are too often prescribed and can become addicting. Vicious cycles occur: Anxiety leads to Substance Dependence, Substance Withdrawal leads to anxiety, and then more substance use ensues.

- **Course.** Unless there is successful intervention, conditioned fears tend to spread gradually, and the patient becomes trapped in an increasingly narrow world. Some patients become completely housebound and can't even tolerate being home alone.

■ 300.23 SOCIAL ANXIETY DISORDER (SOCIAL PHOBIA)

Screening Question

"Do you frequently avoid social situations because you are afraid of doing something stupid or looking silly?"

Diagnostic Prototype

She dreads being with people because she feels so socially inept. She is always afraid that she will do or say something dumb, or that she is not dressed just right or her hair is not in place. And she rejects and humiliates herself with a harshness that could never be duplicated even by the most mean-spirited of external critics. She fears that people are judging her every move harshly, that she will spill the wine, or that she will make a fool of herself on the dance floor. This painful self-consciousness makes her hypervigilantly self-critical, with an attention to tiny details or flaws that could not possibly ever be matched by any outside observer.

Typically feared social situations in Social Anxiety Disorder include talking to strangers; going on a date or to a party; being observed eating, drinking, writing, or going to the bathroom; working with others on a joint project; or giving a speech. These activities are avoided altogether or are endured with mounting dread.

Differential Diagnosis: Rule These Conditions Out

- **Normal shyness.** A survey showed that, next to death, the thing people most feared was going to a party where they didn't know anybody.
- **Agoraphobia.** Avoidance is generalized, not restricted to social situations.
- **Specific Phobia.** A specific object or nonsocial situation is avoided.
- **PTSD or Acute Stress Disorder.** The person avoids reminders of the traumatic event.

- **Separation Anxiety Disorder.** Avoidance is motivated by fears of being separated from a parent or caregiver.
- **OCD.** Situations that trigger compulsive rituals are avoided.
- **Autism Spectrum Disorder,** or **Schizotypal or Schizoid Personality Disorder.** The person lacks interest in other people.
- **Avoidant Personality Disorder.** Avoidance of social situations has an early onset, is long-standing, and is a pervasive pattern of behavior.
- **Major Depressive Disorder.** Loss of interest, pleasure, and energy cause withdrawal from social situations.
- **Psychotic Disorders.** The fears motivating avoidance are delusional.
- **Substance Dependence.** Intoxication and lack of motivation cause social avoidance.
- **Medical illness.** The person avoids the embarrassment of showing some aspect of being sick (e.g., baldness in a patient with cancer, or tremors in someone with Parkinson's disease).

Diagnostic Tips

- **Normal shyness.** It is perfectly normal and acceptable to be shy, easily embarrassed, and fearful of humiliation. This is part of the human condition.
- **Clinical significance.** There is no clear boundary between normal social fears and Social Anxiety Disorder. For the mental disorder to be diagnosed, the symptoms must be severe enough to cause considerable distress or serious limitations in the person's life.
- **Cultural factors.** What is appropriate modesty in Japan might be considered socially avoidant in the United States. What is normal extroversion in the United States might be considered brashness and bad manners in Japan. Compare individuals to their own culture, not yours.
- **Gender.** In many cultures, shyness is encouraged more (or at least discouraged less) in females. Don't confuse this with mental disorder.
- **Single symptom.** Some people have just one social situation that terrifies them. Most common is the fear of public speaking, but the avoidance may be directed toward doing other things in a public place (e.g., eating, writing a check, or going to the bathroom). Usually the impairment doesn't rise to clinical significance, and the person just works around it. But it can sometimes be career-threatening—for example, if

a teacher can't teach lessons or a businessman can't do necessary business lunches.

- **Generalized social anxiety.** In some people, the avoidance generalizes to most or all social contacts. When this has an early onset, it is indistinguishable from Avoidant Personality Disorder.
- **Comorbid Depressive Disorders.** Many people with Social Anxiety Disorder also become secondarily demoralized or depressed.
- **Substance use.** Social anxiety and substance misuse are closely linked. Alcohol is a great social lubricant that dissolves social inhibitions. But using substances for self-medication can get out of hand and evolve into Substance Dependence. Anxiolytic medications (which are too often prescribed) are themselves frequently addicting. As with Agoraphobia, vicious cycles can occur: Anxiety leads to Substance Dependence, Substance Withdrawal leads to anxiety, and more substance use ensues.

■ 300.29 SPECIFIC PHOBIA

Screening Question

"Do you have a particular fear that causes you special trouble, like flying, heights, closed places, animals, seeing blood, or getting an injection?"

Diagnostic Prototype

People with Specific Phobia have an enduring and unreasonable fear of a specific object (like dogs, spiders, or snakes) or a specific situation (like being in a high place, riding in an elevator or airplane, or getting a shot). They either avoid the thing they are afraid of or endure it with intense anxiety and reluctance.

Differential Diagnosis: Rule These Conditions Out

- **Fears that are part of normal life and don't cause much trouble.**
- **Social Anxiety Disorder (Social Phobia).** This is a fear of one or more social situations.
- **Agoraphobia.** This is a phobia of many situations.

- **PTSD or Acute Stress Disorder.** The person fears cues resembling the previously experienced terrible event.
- **Separation Anxiety Disorder.** The individual fears being separated from a caregiver.
- **OCD.** The person fears situations that might trigger compulsive cleaning rituals.

Diagnostic Tips

- **Avoiding overdiagnosis.** Having irrational fears is a ubiquitous part of normal life. Evolution has wired into our brains inborn tendencies to fear things that would be dangerous for us. Chimps and children are afraid of snakes, even if they've never had a chance to learn through bad experiences. Evolution isn't perfect and sometimes overshoots a bit.
- **Clinical significance.** Everyone has at least a few exaggerated fears about something. Most people manage to circumvent them without great distress or impairment in a way that does not count as a mental disorder. For a resident of New York City, having a phobia of snakes is irrelevant to daily functioning; for a farmer in India, it is a whole different story. Specific Phobia should be diagnosed only when the fear and avoidance occur in an important context and have reached a severity and persistence that significantly interfere with the person's life (e.g., a window cleaner is afraid of heights, a medical student faints at the sight of blood, or a truck driver is afraid of bridges).
- **Rates.** The prevalence of Specific Phobia is wildly inflated in epidemiological studies because this kind of research is unable to evaluate clinical significance. Specific Phobias are seen only rarely in clinical practice, most commonly fear of flying. For the most part, people prefer adjusting their lives to accommodate the fear.

■ 300.02 GENERALIZED ANXIETY DISORDER

Screening Questions

"Are you a 'worry-wart,' unnecessarily anxious all the time about a lot of different things?"

Diagnostic Prototype

For those with Generalized Anxiety Disorder, their minds can never rest. All of life's many typical challenges are ready grist for the worry mill—family, finances, health, work, school, friendships, the future, and on and on. The worrying can be accompanied by all sorts of other cognitive symptoms (poor concentration, catastrophization, indecision); mood symptoms (irritability, demoralization); and physical symptoms (nausea, diarrhea, headaches, sweating, shaking, tense muscles, and sleeplessness). The anxiety causes much distress and has a markedly detrimental effect on these persons' daily lives. They seek constant reassurance from others, but never feel really reassured.

CAUTION:
Overdiagnosis of Generalized Anxiety Disorder

In my view, the DSM-5 definition of Generalized Anxiety Disorder is too loose both in the required number of symptoms and in their duration. It is likely to result in the overdiagnosis of the "worried well." Instead, I recommend that this diagnosis be reserved for people whose worries are extensive, pervasive, beyond the ordinary, disabling, enduring (for at least 6 months or more), and not better accounted for by another diagnosis.

Differential Diagnosis:
Rule These Conditions Out

- **Realistic worries.** These require no diagnosis.
- **Adjustment Disorder.** The worries are exaggerated and impairing, but are usually transient and related to a specific realistic stress.
- **Panic Disorder.** The worry is focused on having a panic attack.
- **Social Anxiety Disorder (Social Phobia).** The worry is confined to being embarrassed in social situations.
- **OCD.** The worry is about an obsession (e.g., being contaminated).
- **Separation Anxiety Disorder.** The worry is about being separated from parents or caregivers.

- **Anorexia Nervosa.** The worry is about gaining weight.
- **Body Dysmorphic Disorder.** The worry is about a perceived defect in physical appearance.
- **Somatic Symptom Disorder.** The worries are focused on bodily symptoms.
- **PTSD and Acute Stress Disorder.** The worry is focused on reminders of a traumatic event.
- **Major Depressive Disorder.** The worry has a depressive theme.
- **Psychotic Disorders.** The worries that are not reality-tested become delusions.
- **Substance-Induced Anxiety Disorder.** The anxiety comes from Substance Intoxication (e.g., with caffeine, stimulants) or Substance Withdrawal (e.g., from alcohol, Xanax, Prozac).
- **Anxiety Disorder Due to Another Medical Condition.** For example, anxiety is caused by hyperthyroidism.

Diagnostic Tips

- **Normal worries.** Anxiety and worrying are inherent and often adaptive parts of the perilous human condition.
- **Avoiding overdiagnosis.** A mental disorder is present only when the anxiety and worrying are unrealistic, extreme, enduring, maladaptive, interfering, and impairing. See the box above.
- **Substance use.** Don't forget that anxiety can be a side effect of medication use or medication withdrawal, and can also be caused by either intoxication with or withdrawal from other substances.
- **Medical illnesses.** Always consider the role of medical conditions (e.g., hyperthyroidism, adrenal tumor, congestive heart failure), especially if the anxiety has a late onset.
- **Looking for a more specific diagnosis.** Make sure that the worry is not caused by another condition. Carefully consider all the possibilities in the long list of differential diagnoses. Generalized Anxiety Disorder should be last in line in your consideration—a residual diagnosis used only after everything else has been ruled out.

■ 293.84 ANXIETY DISORDER DUE TO ANOTHER MEDICAL CONDITION (INDICATE THE MEDICAL CONDITION)

Screening Question

"Have you had symptoms of anxiety in association with a medical condition, like an overactive thyroid?"

Diagnostic Prototype

The person's distressing anxiety or panic attacks are directly caused by a medical illness.

Differential Diagnosis: Rule These Conditions Out

- **Adjustment Disorder With Anxiety.** Here, the causal relationship between the medical condition and the symptoms of anxiety is psychologically mediated, not a direct physical result of the illness. For example, the person is anxious about having been diagnosed with a cancer; the cancer itself is not causing anxiety by secreting a hormone.
- **Substance-Induced Anxiety Disorder.** The anxiety is due to a side effect of a medication or other substance.
- **A primary Anxiety Disorder.** The anxiety precedes the substance use or persists for an extended period after it.

Diagnostic Tips

- **A tough diagnosis.** Establishing that a medical condition is directly causing the anxiety can be challenging. The following factors support a direct causal relationship.
- **Onset.** The anxiety symptoms begin simultaneously with, or shortly after, the onset of the medical condition.
- **Linkage.** There is a close relationship between the severity of the anxiety symptoms and the severity of the medical condition—for example, worsening of anxiety symptoms with increasingly high thyroid level in hyperthyroidism.

- **Remission.** The anxiety symptoms resolve with successful treatment of the medical condition.
- **Typicality.** There is evidence from the clinical literature that the medical condition in question is known to cause anxiety symptoms in some individuals.

■ SUBSTANCE-INDUCED ANXIETY DISORDER

291.89 If Alcohol-Induced

292.89 If Induced by Any Other Substance (Indicate Substance)

Screening Question

"Have you had a lot of anxiety symptoms associated with using drugs, drinking alcohol or coffee, taking a medication, or withdrawing from drugs or medication?"

Diagnostic Prototype

Anxiety or panic attacks often occur as a result of taking a substance or medication or withdrawing from it.

Differential Diagnosis: Rule These Conditions Out

- **Anxiety Disorder Due to Another Medical Condition.** The anxiety comes from the medical condition, rather than the medication used to treat it.
- **A primary Anxiety Disorder.** The anxiety precedes the substance use or persists for an extended period after it.
- **Simple Intoxication or Withdrawal.** The anxiety is not out of proportion to what is expected in severity or duration.

Diagnostic Tips

- **Another tough diagnosis.** Establishing that a substance is causing the anxiety can be especially challenging because so many anxious people use substances to self-medicate. The following temporal factors provide clues.
- **Onset.** The anxiety symptoms start *after* the substance use and (ideally) remit shortly after the substance is stopped.
- **Remission.** The anxiety goes away if the person stops using the substance and completes a reasonable period of withdrawal.

■ 300.00 UNSPECIFIED ANXIETY DISORDER

Use the diagnosis of Unspecified Anxiety Disorder when you have determined that there is an anxiety disorder, but there is not enough information to distinguish which one best fits. Often it takes the passage of time and several visits to determine the possible impact of substances or medical illness. This category would also be used for anxiety symptoms that don't resemble any of the specific categories described above but still cause clinically significant distress or impairment.

CHAPTER 6

■ Obsessive–Compulsive
and Related Disorders

IN THIS CHAPTER:

- Obsessive–Compulsive Disorder
- Body Dysmorphic Disorder
- Hoarding Disorder
- Tic Disorders
- Hair-Pulling Disorder (Trichotillomania)
- Substance-Induced Obsessive–Compulsive or Related Disorder
- Obsessive–Compulsive or Related Disorder Due to Another Medical Condition (Indicate the Medical Condition)
- Unspecified Obsessive–Compulsive or Related Disorder

■ 303.3 OBSESSIVE–COMPULSIVE DISORDER

Screening Questions

For obsessions: "Do you ever have weird thoughts that you can't get out of your mind?"

For compulsions: "Are there rituals you can't resist doing over and over and over and over again?"

Diagnostic Prototype

People with OCD have both "obsessions" (intrusive thoughts and images accompanied by anxiety) and "compulsions" (repetitive actions or thoughts that help neutralize the obsessions). A typical obsession is the recurring, persisting, annoying, and irresistible thought "There are dangerous germs everywhere, and I am being contaminated by them." The person knows that her preoccupation with germs far exceeds all reasonable risk, but the obsessive thought has taken on a life of its own and is no longer amenable to logical correction or cognitive control. The only way to reduce the sting of the obsession is to counter it over and over again with a neutralizing compulsion.

Each person discovers a particular ritual that works best for him, and this becomes deeply ingrained and constantly repeated. Usually the compulsion is performed according to rigid rules (e.g., scrubbing the right hand exactly 10 times, then the left 10 times, then the right 10 times, and so on for 100 repetitions while washing with a specific soap, using a specific sink, and drying with a specific towel). If every part of the ritual isn't done just right, it has to be repeated from scratch. This often gets elaborated over time, so that increasing parts of the day are captured.

To keep contamination fears at bay, one person may engage in repeated handwashing; another may take marathon showers; a third may constantly apply a hand sanitizer; a fourth may repetitively scrub the bathroom; and so on. Some people develop cognitive compulsions—for instance, constantly thinking the word "clean" and then spelling it out for 1,000 repetitions; or saying the Lord's Prayer over and over; or counting forward and backward from 1,000. Each person creates a set of personalized rituals that provide no real protection from germs but do manage to reduce the anxiety about being contaminated by them.

Particular obsessions tend to be paired with particular compulsions. The obsessive image of having run over one's child when backing out of the driveway will be linked with the ritual of driving back to the driveway 10 times to check for blood on the asphalt. The repeated impulse to strangle one's quietly sleeping infant will be paired with setting an alarm at hourly intervals throughout the night to check that she is not dead. The obsessive thought that things are out of control will be paired with the ordering ritual of creating and perfecting endless spreadsheets of things to do, inventories, lists of birthdays and favorite foods of all acquaintances, and so on. Obsessions and compulsions are locked in a kind of arms race: The more intense and persistent the obsession and its accompanying anxiety, the more intense and persistent must be the neutralizing compulsion. The pattern causes upset, consumes inordinate time and energy, and interferes with the rest of the person's life. (Note how long the description above is—an illustration of compulsive detail in an attempt to neutralize the obsessive fear of being incomplete.)

Differential Diagnosis: Rule These Conditions Out

- **Normal obsessions and rituals of everyday life.** We all have some.

Other Conditions Characterized by Recurrent Intrusive Thoughts

- **Major Depressive Disorder.** Depressive preoccupations.
- **Body Dysmorphic Disorder.** Intrusive thoughts that a body part is horribly ugly.
- **Generalized Anxiety Disorder.** Excessive but realistic worries about everyday things.
- **PTSD or Acute Stress Disorder.** Repetitive memories of the terrible event.
- **Anorexia Nervosa.** Preoccupations about being fat.
- **Substance Dependence.** Intrusive cravings and thoughts about a drug or alcohol.
- **Paraphilic Disorders.** Intrusive sexual thoughts.
- **Delusional Disorder.** Obsessions that have turned into delusions (e.g., "I will die because of the contamination, and nothing I do can stop it").
- **Schizotypal Personality Disorder.** Odd, eccentric thoughts, but not experienced as externally driven and intrusive.
- **Somatic Symptom Disorder.** Intrusive worries about having a serious illness.

Other Conditions Characterized by Repetitive Behaviors
That Are Experienced as Outside One's Control

- **Hair-Pulling Disorder (Trichotillomania).** Repeated need to pull hair.
- **Tic Disorders.** Repeated stereotyped motor movements or vocalizations.
- **Substance Dependence.** Repeated urge to use substances despite harmful effects.
- **Bulimia Nervosa.** Repeated binges and purges.
- **Hoarding.** Compulsive collecting.
- **Autism Spectrum Disorder.** Stereotyped rituals.
- **Schizophrenia.** Bizarre, disorganized behavior.
- **Obsessive–Compulsive Personality Disorder.** Rigid, perfectionistic behavior, but no true obsessions or compulsions.

Diagnostic Tips

- **Obsessions and rituals as often adaptive parts of life.** Don't diagnose OCD if obsessions and rituals are harmless, prudent, or part of a cultural or religious practice. It may make sense (and does no harm) to check twice or even three times to make sure the front door is locked or the oven is off. Praying 2 hours a day is a religious observance rather than a symptom if it is expected by the person's religious community; it is symptom only when it is an individual and idiosyncratic reaction to an obsession.
- **Intrusive thoughts: Obsessions or cognitive compulsions?** It depends on how they function. Repetitive unwanted thoughts are classified as obsessions if they are accompanied by anxiety, but as compulsions if they reduce anxiety. The distinction is important because there are different implications. Compulsions are much easier than obsessions to treat by exposure techniques.
- **Levels of insight.** Some patients with OCD have good insight, some poor, some none. Having good insight doesn't mean that patients can stop an intrusive, anxiety-producing thought or the ritual needed to neutralize it; it just means that they know it doesn't make any sense and that the whole business feels ego-alien. For example, a patient's obsessions with contamination may seem completely weird and dumb to her,

but she feels extremely nervous unless she keeps washing her hands, since this calms her anxiety. Another keeps at it until his hands are painfully red and raw because having hurt hands is better than feeling so nervous (even though he knows it is silly to be so worried about contamination, and self-destructive to be washing all the time). Patients can't stop or control the behaviors, despite their clear awareness of their utter senselessness. This is what is meant by "good insight." At the opposite extreme is "no insight." These patients will argue with great conviction and reams of scientific papers that dangerous germs are indeed lurking everywhere in the environment. They assert that you are crazy for not being equally concerned, and are convinced that having raw hands beats having dangerous germs on their bodies. "Poor insight" is somewhere in between and may fluctuate from "good insight" to "no insight," depending on clinical status, situation, stress, and response to treatment. Useful questions to test insight are these: "How sure are you that all this makes sense and that the gain is worth the pain? 100%? 50%? 25%? Not convinced at all? Would you stop washing if you could?"

- **Relation to Delusional Disorder.** Sometimes the lack of insight is so profound and the intrusive thoughts so bizarre that the patient approaches or crosses the fuzzy boundary between severe obsession and Delusional Disorder (e.g., a man who prays 20 hours every day to wipe out the obsessive thought that not praying will kill his child). Delusional OCD requires medication treatment in addition to cognitive-behavioral therapy.

- **Relation to Schizotypal Personality Disorder.** About 5% of patients with OCD have preexisting Schizotypal Personality Disorder. They are particularly likely to have the "no insight" or delusional form of OCD and to be more difficult to treat.

- **Relation to Obsessive–Compulsive Personality Disorder.** OCD and Obsessive–Compulsive Personality Disorder share a name; they do sometimes occur together; and both may be diagnosed if both are present. But they are fundamentally different. Most people with OCD don't have Obsessive–Compulsive Personality Disorder, and vice versa.

- **Embarrassment.** Patients, especially those with good insight, will withhold or minimize the extent and strangeness of their obsessions—

particularly if these are sexual ("You are a whore"), violent ("Kill your baby"), or sacrilegious ("Screw God").

■ 300.7 BODY DYSMORPHIC DISORDER

Screening Question

"Are you comfortable with your physical appearance?"

Diagnostic Prototype

People with Body Dysmorphic Disorder have disproportionate concerns about a real or imagined flaw in the way they look (e.g., "My nose is way too big," "My breasts are way too small," "My abs are way too flabby"). They may spend endless hours in front of a mirror, or may do everything possible to avoid ever being near a mirror. The imagined or exaggerated defect takes on greater and greater significance and can come to rule all life decisions, causing increasing constriction in social relations and work. At first, they give up parties and dating because they can't stand the thought of what others are thinking about their "hideous" appearance. Then they give up their jobs because they can't stand the imagined glances and smirks of coworkers. At the extreme, a patient may be trapped in her own house, able to go out only after midnight disguised in a loose trenchcoat, wrap-around sunglasses, and a wide-brimmed hat that covers her face.

Differential Diagnosis: Rule These Conditions Out

- **Normal disappointments in appearance.** Everyone has these.
- **Anorexia Nervosa.** The person's concerns are restricted to feeling fat.
- **Gender Dysphoria.** The concerns are restricted to feeling that one's body is discordant with one's gender identity.
- **Social Anxiety Disorder (Social Phobia).** Avoidance of social situations is not so exclusively focused on embarrassment about physical appearance.

- **Major Depressive Disorder.** Dissatisfaction with self is not focused on a physical defect.
- **Delusional Disorder.** The body preoccupation is bizarre, is held with delusional intensity, and causes great impairment.

Diagnostic Tips

- **Normal self-loathing.** It is not really normal for anyone to be completely satisfied with body appearance; part of human nature is to find something wrong in the mirror and to wish there were an easy fix.
- **Clinically significant impairment.** This can take various forms: inordinate time spent checking the defect, frantic efforts to conceal it, futile attempts at corrective plastic surgery, and/or the avoidance of necessary social and work activities.
- **Reassurance.** This provides little (if any) and only temporary relief.
- **Which flaws?** People are most self-conscious about real or imagined defects in facial appearance, but other parts of the body may become the focus, particularly those related to secondary sexual characteristics.
- **Levels of insight.** As in OCD, some patients with Body Dysmorphic Disorder have good insight, some poor, some none. Insight may or may not protect them from the extremes of self-loathing, but it does reduce the risks of complete social avoidance and disfiguring plastic surgery.
- **Relation to somatic delusions.** The concerns may over time become increasingly intense, fixed, and bizarre, and may lead to disastrous consequences. The boundary between "no insight" and "somatic delusions" is fuzzy and drawn differently by different evaluators.
- **Plastic surgery.** The person may pursue repeated cosmetic procedures with a cumulatively negative impact on appearance. This can make matters much worse by providing new and better targets for critical self-examination, preoccupation, attempts at disguise, avoidance, and additional plastic surgery.
- **Malpractice suits.** People with Body Dysmorphic Disorder are a plastic surgeon's worst nightmare. They can rarely achieve a successful external fix of an internally driven dissatisfaction, but often lack the

insight to own the problem. Instead, they blame the surgeon's lack of skill.

- **Embarrassment.** Patients are often exquisitely embarrassed about their embarrassment. Informants are helpful.

■ 300.3 HOARDING DISORDER

Screening Question

"Do you find it impossible to ever throw anything out?"

Diagnostic Prototype

A person with Hoarding Disorder can't bear to part with any object, even completely worthless ones. His house is a cluttered labyrinth of old newspapers, plastic milk cartons, torn clothing, broken appliances, his third-grade catcher's mitt, three sets of the World Book Encyclopedia, four broken bicycles, and many thousands each of videotapes, record albums, paperbacks, and old calendars. He can't get into his garage, and many rooms in his house are little caves carved out of mountains of stuff. His friends and neighbors complain that he has created a health and fire hazard. He completely agrees and is very embarrassed, but gets too anxious to continue whenever he tries to throw anything out. He is fully aware that it is a very bad idea to keep adding to the mound, but he can't control the impulse to do so.

Differential Diagnosis: Rule These Conditions Out

- **OCD.** The clutter results from an obsession (e.g., the person does not throw out old shoes because of contamination fears about touching them).
- **Major Depressive Disorder.** The clutter is a consequence of the person's being slowed down or indifferent.
- **Schizophrenia.** The clutter comes from a delusion (e.g., the person fills the room with papers as a buffer to "alien rays," or as a result of general disorganization and bizarre behavior).

- **Major Neurocognitive Disorder (Dementia).** The person has poor judgment and is too disorganized to get rid of things.
- **Autism Spectrum Disorder.** Collecting is a manifestation of stereotyped and restricted interests (e.g., collecting old train schedules).

Diagnostic Tips

- **Normal "pack rat" behavior.** Not all hoarding or sloppiness constitutes a mental disorder. The hoarding must be severe and distressing, must cause impairment, or must be a health hazard.
- **Insight.** People rarely self-refer for hoarding. A patient's partner is much more likely to have reached the limit of tolerance and will be a much better informant about the extent of the problem.
- **Embarrassment.** Patients will often not volunteer information about this disorder unless asked.
- **A new disorder.** Hoarding used to be considered an aspect of OCD, but has been separated out because it appears to have different brain mechanisms and treatment implications.

■ TIC DISORDERS

307.23 Tourette's Disorder

307.22 Chronic Motor or Vocal Tic Disorder

307.21 Provisional Tic Disorder

333.3 Substance-Induced Tic Disorder (Indicate Substance)

333.3 Tic Disorder Due to Another Medical Condition (Indicate the Medical Condition)

307.20 Unspecified Tic Disorder

Screening Questions

For a parent: "Does your child move or make sounds that he can't control?"

For an adult patient: "Do you move or make sounds that you can't control?"

Diagnostic Prototype

The person suddenly and irresistibly makes a rapid, recurrent, and stereo-typed movement or vocalization. The most common motor tics are blinking, shrugging, or grimacing. The most common verbal tics are grunting and coughing, although rarely there may be uttering of obscene words or phrases.

Diagnostic Tips

- **Coding.** The primary Tic Disorders differ only in the extent and duration of the clinical presentation. The fact that they have separate names and codes does not mean that they are separate disorders. They probably just represent course and severity variants of one disorder. It probably would be better to have one Tic Disorder with different subtypes, but we are stuck with their being artificially split apart.
- **Tourette's Disorder.** This is the most severe form, requiring multiple verbal and motor tics occurring regularly and often over a year or more.
- **Chronic Motor or Vocal Tic Disorder.** The code for this should be used when there are either vocal or motor tics but not both.
- **Provisional Tic Disorder.** The code for this should be used if duration is less than 1 year.
- **Characteristics.** Although tics feel irresistible, the person can usually suppress them for a period of time and may learn ways of disguising them. Age of onset is usually early in life and almost always before age 18.
- **Relation to OCD.** People with Tourette's Disorder are at increased risk for OCD symptoms, which often have an early onset and poorer response to treatment than in uncomplicated OCD. This presentation may be related to streptococcal infections (see the section below on OCD symptoms due to medical illness).
- **Relation to ADHD.** Ask about hyperactivity, impulsivity, and distractibility, since these symptoms are common in conjunction with Tourette's Disorder. Also note that stimulants can increase the severity of tics.
- **Social withdrawal.** This may occur secondary to teasing and embarrassment.

■ 312.39 HAIR-PULLING DISORDER (TRICHOTILLOMANIA)

Screening Question

"Do you pull out your hair?"

Diagnostic Prototype

The person feels an irresistible urge to pull out hair, most commonly from the scalp, eyebrows, and eyelashes. There is a sense of relief once this is done, but it is accompanied by anxiety to disguise the results. Hair pulling usually occurs when the person is alone, bored, or under stress, but may also be done furtively in public.

Differential Diagnosis: Rule These Conditions Out

- **Medical causes of alopecia.**
- **Normal hair pulling.** Hair pulling can be a temporary habit in children, or normal in adults if it doesn't cause distress or impairment.
- **Other mental disorders.** For example, hair pulling may be a response to a delusion in a Psychotic Disorder.

Diagnostic Tip

- **Embarrassment.** People are usually very embarrassed about Hair-Pulling Disorder. If you don't see evidence of it, you probably won't hear about it.

■ 292.9 SUBSTANCE-INDUCED OBSESSIVE–COMPULSIVE OR RELATED DISORDER

OCD symptoms and tics sometimes occur, especially in people using stimulants or cocaine.

■ 293.84 OBSESSIVE–COMPULSIVE OR RELATED DISORDER DUE TO ANOTHER MEDICAL CONDITION (INDICATE THE MEDICAL CONDITION)

Two conditions are of special interest here:

• **Pediatric autoimmune neuropsychiatric disorders associated with streptococcal infection (PANDAS).** This describes the rapid, intense onset of OCD symptoms and/or tics caused by a streptococcal infection (strep throat or scarlet fever). PANDAS generally occur in prepubescent children. Prompt clinical evaluation, laboratory testing, diagnosis, and antibiotic treatment are essential to reduce the severity of resulting OCD and tic symptoms.

• **Pediatric acute-onset neuropsychiatric syndrome (PANS).** This is a broader term that includes all abrupt-onset OCD in children, not just those related to strep infection.

■ 300.00 UNSPECIFIED OBSESSIVE–COMPULSIVE OR RELATED DISORDER

Use the Unspecified code when you have determined that there is a problem that resembles those described in this chapter but it doesn't fit well within any of them, or when there is not enough information to distinguish whether an infection or other medical illness has played a causal role.

CHAPTER 7

■ Trauma- and Stressor-Related Disorders

IN THIS CHAPTER:

- ■ Posttraumatic Stress Disorder
- ■ CAUTION: The Stressor Gatekeeper
- ■ Acute Stress Disorder
- ■ Unspecified Trauma- or Stressor-Related Disorder
- ■ Adjustment Disorder

■ 309.81 POSTTRAUMATIC STRESS DISORDER

Screening Question

"Have you experienced a traumatic event that keeps haunting you in terrible memories, flashbacks, or nightmares?"

Diagnostic Prototype

PTSD applies only if someone has suffered through an unusually dreadful trauma (e.g., witnessing or being threatened with violent death, suffering serious injury, or being raped). It is a sad statement that the stressors most likely to cause PTSD are those that are inflicted deliberately by human beings (e.g., combat, rape, torture, battery). Other qualifying catastrophes include accidents, hurricanes, earthquakes, fires, and floods. The most characteristic PTSD symptoms are intrusive daytime memories, images, or flashbacks of the gruesome details of what happened. Fearsome and repetitive nightmares vividly replay the tragedy at night. Cues that are in any way (even remotely) reminiscent of the event may have to be carefully avoided, lest they trigger a renewal of terror and its concomitant physical symptoms. The person may distrust others and lose any faith in the future ("I am cursed; nothing will ever be right again"). Numb and detached, he finds life and relationships flat and meaningless. The person has trouble sleeping and concentrating; he is jumpy, irritable, and easily startled. Easily angered, those with PTSD may also be angry at themselves and feel guilty for surviving. Most persons with PTSD begin having symptoms shortly after the event, but some experience a delayed response that begins months or even years later, perhaps when they are confronted by a reminder of the dreaded event or by a new source of stress.

CAUTION: The Stressor Gatekeeper

The only definitional hurdle that protects against the inappropriate forensic diagnosis of PTSD is the requirement that the patient must have had an intense contact with an unusually severe stressor. DSM-5 lowers this threshold considerably by allowing the diagnosis of PTSD in people who have had no direct exposure, but have merely learned about a violent, traumatic event that was experienced by a close relative or friend. This may make good clinical sense, but it inadvertently creates a forensic disaster: All of the victim's relatives and friends can now claim damages based on their secondhand PTSD.

I recommend that in forensic proceedings, the diagnosis be used only when the person has had direct experience of the traumatic stressor.

Differential Diagnosis: Rule These Conditions Out

- **PTSD symptoms without PTSD.** Typical PTSD symptoms are present, but not at a level sufficient to cause clinically significant distress or impairment.
- **Acute Stress Disorder.** Symptoms are confined to the first month after experiencing the stressor.
- **Adjustment Disorder.** Like PTSD, this is a reaction to stress, but either the stressor is not extreme enough or the symptomatic reaction to it is subthreshold.

- **Another mental disorder.** The reaction to the extreme stressor is a Depressive Disorder, an Anxiety Disorder, or Brief Psychotic Disorder, not the characteristic symptoms of PTSD.

- **Other causes of flashbacks.** For example, the perceptual distortions come from substance use, head injury, a Bipolar or Depressive Disorder, or a Psychotic Disorder.

- **Malingering.** This is especially likely when the stressor is marginal and/or there is financial or other gain from having a diagnosis of PTSD.

Diagnostic Tips

- **The requirement of an extreme stressor.** Merely severe life stressors—such as the expectable loss of a loved one, divorce, being fired from a job, or failing out of school—don't count.

- **Symptom severity.** Almost everyone will have some symptoms that resemble PTSD after being confronted by an extreme stressor. These are normal and completely expectable reactions to terrible events. To count as PTSD, the symptoms must be severe and persistent, and must also cause clinically significant distress or impairment.

- **Durations.** Acute Stress Disorder applies to symptoms occurring during a period of 3 days to 1 month after the stressor. PTSD, Acute applies to the period between 1 and 3 months. PTSD, Chronic applies to PTSD that lasts longer than 3 months. PTSD, With Delayed Onset describes symptoms that have their onset more than 6 months after the occurrence of the stressor.

- **Importance of PTSD in forensics.** The presence or absence of PTSD is often a central issue in civil lawsuits because it can be a big contributor to the level of damages awarded to trauma victims. PTSD is also a major factor in disability claims (especially in the military, but also often in civilian life).

- **Forensic problem.** PTSD is one of the most difficult of all psychiatric diagnoses to evaluate in forensic contexts. The symptoms are completely subjective, are easy to fake or exaggerate, and carry potentially huge gain. At the other extreme, some people with PTSD stoically deny what are quite obvious symptoms.

■ 308.3 ACUTE STRESS DISORDER

Screening Question

"Have you experienced a traumatic event that keeps haunting you in terrible memories, flashbacks, or nightmares?"

Diagnostic Prototype

Acute Stress Disorder is equivalent to the clinical presentation of PTSD in every way except for its short duration—below 1 month. Acute Stress Disorder is the early form of PTSD. It requires that the individual had experienced the same types of extreme stressors and had exactly the same types of symptom presentation. Acute Stress Disorder should not be used if a person has symptoms without clinically significant distress or impairment.

Some people with Acute Stress Disorder recover from it; others have persistent, clinically significant symptoms and eventually qualify for the diagnosis of PTSD.

■ 309.89 UNSPECIFIED TRAUMA- OR STRESSOR-RELATED DISORDER

The diagnosis of Unspecified Trauma- or Stressor-Related Disorder can be used in clinical situations when the stressor is not extreme enough to qualify for PTSD but classic symptoms are present, or when the stressor is extreme enough but the symptom criteria are not met. I caution that this is not a reliable diagnosis and should not be taken seriously in forensic proceedings. It is included only for clinical use.

■ ADJUSTMENT DISORDER

309.0   Adjustment Disorder With Depressed Mood

309.24 Adjustment Disorder With Anxiety

**309.28 Adjustment Disorder With Mixed Anxiety/
          Depressed Mood**

309.3   Adjustment Disorder With Conduct Disturbance

**309.4   Adjustment Disorder With Mixed Disturbance of
          Emotions and Conduct**

309.9   Unspecified Adjustment Disorder

Screening Question

"Are you having problems dealing with the stresses in your life?"

Diagnostic Prototype

In response to a life stress, the person has symptoms that cause clinically significant distress or impairment, but aren't severe enough to fit any of the mental disorders described elsewhere.

Differential Diagnosis: Rule These Conditions Out

- **A normal reaction to stress.** The symptoms are within expectable limits and don't cause clinically significant distress or impairment. See Chapter 18 if a diagnostic code is necessary.
- **Bereavement.** This is not to be considered a mental disorder.
- **Another mental disorder.** Any diagnosis that is more specific than Adjustment Disorder takes precedence over it.

Diagnostic Tips

- **Adjustment Disorder as a residual category.** It is not meant to be used if the response to stress fits one of the more specific diagnoses covered above.
- **Adjustment Disorder as a mental disorder.** It is not suitable for people who are having no more than expectable symptoms in response to a difficult life stress. Don't diagnose mental disorder if someone is doing

well enough in dealing with the stress and lacks clinically significant distress or impairment.

- **The requirement of an external stress.** It is not Adjustment Disorder if there is no stress to be adjusting to.
- **Instability of the diagnosis.** Most often Adjustment Disorder is self-limited. Sometimes it evolves into a more specific mental disorder.
- **Chronic Adjustment Disorder.** This can occur if the stress is chronic (e.g., a difficult job or marriage, constant financial trouble) and the symptoms persist for many months or years in response to it.

CHAPTER 8

■ Schizophrenia Spectrum and Other Psychotic Disorders

IN THIS CHAPTER:

- Schizophrenia
- Schizophreniform Disorder
- Schizoaffective Disorder
- Delusional Disorder
- Shared Psychotic Disorder (Folie à Deux)
- Brief Psychotic Disorder
- Substance-Induced Psychotic Disorder
- Psychotic Disorder Due to Another Medical Condition (Indicate the Medical Condition)
- Catatonic Disorder Due to Another Medical Condition (Indicate the Medical Condition)
- Unspecified Psychotic Disorder
- CAUTION: Attenuated Psychosis Syndrome

■ 295.9 SCHIZOPHRENIA

Screening Question

"Do you ever hear voices, believe that people mean to harm you, or lose touch with reality?"

Diagnostic Prototype

There really isn't a uniform prototype for Schizophrenia because it presents so variably and overlaps with so many other disorders. The symptom pattern consists of some combination of "psychotic symptoms" (e.g., delusions and hallucinations); "disorganization" (e.g., thought disorder and bizarre behavior); and "negative symptoms" (e.g., a poverty in emotional life, motivation, thought, and relationships). None of the various symptoms that define Schizophrenia is specific to Schizophrenia; they all occur in many other mental disorders that can be confused with it. And none of the symptoms that define Schizophrenia is pathognomonic of, or always present in, Schizophrenia. There are some patients who present with the complete package, but most have only varying pieces of it.

The onset and course are also variable. Emil Kraepelin's classic description featured an early onset during adolescence, a chronic course throughout the lifespan, and frequent deterioration. In current usage, the term Schizophrenia can cover onsets throughout the life cycle and have a much more favorable outcome in a sizable minority of patients.

So we are faced with a diagnostic paradox: Two patients bearing the label Schizophrenia may look very different from each other, while a patient with Schizophrenia may be hard to distinguish from patients with the other disorders that can cause psychosis (e.g., Bipolar or Depressive Disorders, Substance-Related Disorders, and medical illness). Classic cases will be unmistakable. But for the common puzzling case, revisit the diagnosis as you get to know the patient better and acquire more data on the longitudinal evolution of symptoms. What you are looking for is the presence of psychosis, disorganization, and negative symptoms, as well as the absence of other etiologies (e.g., a Bipolar or Depressive Disorder, a Substance-Related Disorder, or a neurological illness).

Differential Diagnosis: Rule These Conditions Out

- **Schizoaffective Disorder.** Mood symptoms are prominent in the overall presentation, but psychotic symptoms persist even when there are no mood episodes.
- **Major Depressive Disorder, Severe With Psychotic Features.** Psychotic symptoms are restricted to the Major Depressive Episodes.
- **Bipolar I Disorder, Severe With Psychotic Features.** Psychotic symptoms are restricted to the Manic or Major Depressive Episodes.

- **Schizotypal Personality Disorder.** There are no psychotic symptoms.
- **Schizophreniform Disorder.** Exactly the same symptoms as those in Schizophrenia are present, but they last for more than 1 month and less than 6 months.
- **Brief Psychotic Disorder.** The same symptoms as in Schizophrenia are present, but they last less than 1 month.
- **Delusional Disorder.** Only delusions are present—no hallucinations, disorganization, or negative symptoms.
- **Substance-Induced Psychotic Disorder.** Delusions or hallucinations occur only during Substance Intoxication or Withdrawal or their immediate aftermath.
- **Psychotic Disorder Due to Another Medical Condition.** Hallucinations or delusions are caused by a medical illness impairing brain function.
- **Autism Spectrum Disorder.** There are no prominent delusions or hallucinations.
- **Shared Psychotic Disorder.** The delusional beliefs are imposed by a dominant partner and then disappear when the two are separated.
- **Malingering.** Consider this if there is something to be gained by "faking crazy" (e.g., avoiding criminal responsibility).
- **Political or religious zealotry.** The person has bizarre beliefs, but these are shared by others.

Diagnostic Tips

- **Problems in defining Schizophrenia.** As noted above, there is no pathognomonic symptom or uniform course; presentations are heterogeneous; and the boundaries with other disorders are fuzzy.
- **The pattern.** Schizophrenia requires a combination of psychotic symptoms, disorganized speech and behavior, negative symptoms, and a chronic course.
- **Defining psychosis.** The term "psychosis" has been used in very different ways. The narrowest definition is hallucinations and delusions without insight or reality testing. A middle definition is any hallucination or delusion, even if the person has developed some insight and reality testing. A loose definition includes as "psychotic" disorganized thought, emotions, and behavior. Schizophrenia was overdiagnosed in

the past (particularly in the United States) when too much reliance was placed on subjective judgments using the looser definition.

- **Diagnosing delusions.** We all hold false beliefs, sometimes quite stubbornly. It is difficult to draw a firm line separating psychotic "delusions" from nonpsychotic "overvalued ideas." The term "delusions" refers only to false beliefs that are idiosyncratic, incredible, impervious to contrary argument, blind to overwhelming disproof, and held with absolute certainty, and that severely impair functioning and contact with consensual reality.

- **Delusions versus religious and political beliefs.** The distinction between delusions and political/religious zealotry comes up as a heated forensic question every time a terrorist commits a mass murder justified by a strange ideology that this was necessary for the greater good (e.g., to maintain racial purity, to stop the tyranny of technology, to protect the one true faith, to begin the apocalypse, and so on). The defense lawyers usually want to plead insanity; the perpetrator finds this an insult to himself and to his cause; and the psychiatrists line up on both sides of the question. There is usually no clear right answer, but be cautious in labeling someone delusional if his beliefs (however foolish or repugnant) are shared by a sizable group, and if the person lacks disorganized and negative symptoms. The terrorist usually deserves what he prefers—prison rather than hospital.

- **"Bizarre" and "nonbizarre" delusions.** Some people suggest that the presence of bizarre delusions might help distinguish Schizophrenia from psychotic Bipolar or Depressive Disorders and Delusional Disorder. There are two problems with this contention. First, the distinction between "bizarre" and "nonbizarre" delusions is too much in the eye of the beholder to be made reliably. Second, bizarre delusions occur more often in Schizophrenia, but are not specific to it; they can also occasionally occur as part of the other disorders discussed in this chapter, in Bipolar or Depressive Disorders, and in Substance Intoxication or medical illness.

- **Diagnosing hallucinations.** Not all strange perceptual experiences are psychotic. Many people have illusions—misperceptions of actual sensory stimuli that are coming from the world (e.g., numerous people are convinced that they have seen alien ships in bright lights shining in the night sky). Illusions are not indicative of psychosis and happen to normal people all the time. By definition, hallucinations are gener-

98 ■ ESSENTIALS OF PSYCHIATRIC DIAGNOSIS

ated internally within the brain in the absence of any sensory stimulus coming from external reality. Studies show that hallucinations are surprisingly common; about 10% of the general population admits to sometimes having them. To be considered psychotic, the hallucinations should occur without insight, at least during part of the illness. Some people can apply reality testing to their hallucinations (i.e., they know they are having an internally generated experience). Auditory hallucinations are most characteristic of Schizophrenia—especially voices that seem to come from outside and talk to each other. But even these are not specific to Schizophrenia and can occur in other forms of psychosis. Other types of hallucinations (visual, tactile, taste, smell) can occur in Schizophrenia, but are much more specific to a substance use or a neurological problem. Somatic hallucinations can also occur, but are difficult to distinguish from real body sensations unless they are bizarre (e.g., "I can feel cosmic rays burning out my liver cells"). Always ask about "command hallucinations" that order the person to do something terrible, often in a peremptory, authoritative, believable, and hard-to-resist way. These can lead to dangerous or aggressive behavior if the person lacks insight and feels he has to obey the voice.

- **Diagnosing disorganized speech (also known as "loosening of associations").** If subjected to microscopic observation, all of us display logical gaps in our speech and thinking. To count toward a diagnosis of Schizophrenia, the speech (and the thought behind it) must be obviously and profoundly disorganized, derailed, and close to incoherent (at least at times). Much of the previous overdiagnosis of Schizophrenia came from an exaggeration of the clinical significance of small and commonplace logical blips. It shouldn't take an expert to judge disorganized speech. If the thinking problems aren't so obvious that everyone can spot them, they probably shouldn't count. By the way, this is the only symptom of Schizophrenia that can't be convincingly faked; its presence is one way of ruling out Malingering.

- **Diagnosing disorganized behavior.** This is tough because lots of people who are eccentric and act strangely do not have Schizophrenia. The behavior has to be so bizarre and disorganized that no one can miss it.

- **Diagnosing negative symptoms.** Although far less dramatic than psychotic or disorganized symptoms, negative symptoms are an important contributor to the impairment of Schizophrenia. Unfortunately, negative symptoms are very difficult to diagnose accurately. They are on a continuum with normality, resemble depression, can be due to drug side effects, and can result from demoralization over the effects of the positive symptoms. Schizophrenia has been overdiagnosed by clinicians who are too ready to diagnose negative symptoms without considering other possible causes.

- **Symptoms versus course.** There has been a historical debate over whether Schizophrenia is better defined by its cross-sectional symptom pattern (à la Bleuler or Schneider) or by its deteriorating course (à la Kraepelin). Neither approach is by itself satisfactory. The cross-sectional symptom pattern is relatively nonspecific and shared by several other disorders, and the course is also neither specific nor nearly so uniformly gloomy as once portrayed. We have to accept that Schizophrenia is necessarily a heterogeneous concept best defined by requiring a combination of characteristic symptoms and a chronic, but not necessarily deteriorating, course. It should be noted, though, that the Bleulerian cross-sectional approach is particularly apt to cause overdiagnosis.

- **First episodes.** First episodes present a diagnostic conundrum of great clinical moment. It is important to identify and treat Schizophrenia early in its course, in order to minimize the overall lifetime burden of illness. But it is also difficult to be accurate in early diagnosis because of the patient's short track record, particularly if he is also using drugs. Always be prepared to revisit initial diagnostic impressions as you learn more about the patient's symptoms and have more information about the course.

■ 295.40 SCHIZOPHRENIFORM DISORDER

Screening Question

"Do you ever hear voices, believe that people mean to harm you, or lose touch with reality?"

Diagnostic Prototype

Schizophreniform Disorder and Schizophrenia are exactly the same in presentation and differ only in duration: Schizophreniform Disorder has to last more than 1 but less than 6 months, and Schizophrenia has to endure for more than 6 months. There is only one reason to make this artificial and arbitrary distinction: Patients who are able to recover more quickly have a better lifetime prognosis. Aside from short duration, the other indicators of good prognosis include normal premorbid personality; absence of prior episodes; acute onset; presence of stressors; possible role of drugs; absence of thought disorder, bizarre behavior, or negative symptoms; and presence of mood symptoms. The differential diagnosis is the same as for Schizophrenia (see above).

■ 295.70 SCHIZOAFFECTIVE DISORDER

Screening Question

"Do you ever hear voices, believe that people mean to harm you, or lose touch with reality? Do you have mood swings?"

Diagnostic Prototype

Schizoaffective Disorder is provided as a boundary diagnosis for patients who don't fit well within either Schizophrenia or a Mood Disorder and have features of both. There is no clear boundary between these disorders. Many patients present with features of each, and genetic studies show great overlap. As in Major Depressive or Bipolar I Disorder, Severe With Psychotic Features, there are episodes of mania and/or depression accompanied by delusions or hallucinations. As in Schizophrenia, there are periods of delusions and/or hallucinations that occur in the absence of mood episodes. Mood symptoms must be a prominent part of the disorder. The differential diagnosis is the same as for Schizophrenia (see above).

◼ 297.1 DELUSIONAL DISORDER

Screening Question

"Do people ever say you have really strange ideas?"

Diagnostic Prototype

The patient has persistent delusions, but doesn't have the other disorganized and negative symptoms that are characteristic of Schizophrenia. There are no hallucinations, no oddities of speech, no bizarre behavior, no emotional blunting, no lost motivation, and no deterioration in the arenas of life that are unrelated to the delusion. Indeed, the person may seem completely normal, charming, and intelligent, so long as anything touching on the delusion is not part of the conversation. Then something triggers the delusion, and the patient expresses startlingly strange beliefs that take a false premise to its illogical conclusion. The delusional belief is fixed, false, and resistant to either rational argument or compelling contrary evidence. But the psychosis can be tightly encapsulated, allowing surprisingly good day-to-day functioning in the other spheres of life. Among the delusional people I have treated were doctors, lawyers, and teachers who appeared to be floridly psychotic when discussing their delusions, but were still able to do their jobs.

People tend to specialize in one or another content of delusion, but mixtures also can occur.

Paranoid delusions weave together a fabric of hidden signs and threats to find evidence of conspiracy and persecution. The person feels singled out for humiliation, harm, or attack; believes she is observed, followed, and controlled by a malevolent opposition; and is constantly vigilant against being cheated, deceived, or discriminated against.

Delusions of jealousy are sometimes combined with persecutory delusions; sometimes they occur independently. Every word, look, gesture, article of dress, chance encounter, or email is misinterpreted and taken as proof positive of the partner's unfaithfulness. The person tortures himself and nags his partner to death with unremitting demands either for a complete confession, for compelling evidence of fidelity, or for both. Repeated protestations of innocence by his partner are futile and instead are somehow twisted to provide yet further confirmation of guilt.

Somatic delusions involve the belief that one or another body part is impaired in some special and unrealistic way, or that the person has an undetermined illness, usually deemed to be fatal. The boundary between somatic delusions and intense hypochondriacal concerns is especially difficult to draw.

Erotomanic delusions are romantic in origin, but frustrating in result. The person believes that someone has fallen in love with her, but that the other person is afraid or unable to declare himself. She sees hidden signs everywhere of his secret love and refuses to accept as valid any evidence to the contrary, including direct disavowals by the intended. What starts as positive feelings can turn bitterly negative with intense disappointment and frustration when the intended fails to deliver on imagined promises.

Grandiose delusions are less common now than they once were. We no longer see many Napoleons, Christs, or people declaring themselves the new Messiah (except pilgrims driven mad by the heady experience of being in Jerusalem).

Differential Diagnosis: Rule These Conditions Out

- **OCD and Body Dysmorphic Disorder.** In their severe forms, both these disorders can be associated with delusions. See Chapter 6.
- **Schizophrenia.** The person has delusions, but also has hallucinations, thought disorder, negative symptoms, and/or bizarre behavior.

Otherwise, follow the same differential diagnosis as for Schizophrenia (see above).

Diagnostic Tips

- **Boundary of delusions.** As mentioned above in the discussion of Schizophrenia, there is no clear boundary demarcating the delusional from the kooky. Strange belief systems are endemic among political and religious fanatics, UFO enthusiasts, cultists, terrorists, and radio talk show hosts. An individual is not considered psychotic unless he is alone in his idiosyncratic beliefs. It is not the wrongness of the belief that defines a delusion, but rather its being held in the face of universal consensual invalidation. Of course, this distinction is difficult to apply and can lead to some strange paradoxes. Galileo might accurately have fit this definition of "delusional," given the consensual state of scientific knowledge in 1600. And Jim Jones might not have been considered delusional, given the fact that his Jonestown cult provided consensual validation of his wacky and dangerous beliefs. Use your best clinical judgment in sorting out this definitional labyrinth.

- **Degree of certainty.** It is useful to assess the certainty and fixity with which the belief is held. "Are you 100% sure, 90%, perhaps 80%? What makes you so sure? What evidence or experiment would prove you right? What could prove you wrong?" It is not usually a good idea to get into a confrontation with the patient over the reality or idiosyncrasy of a delusional belief, but it is important to determine the degree to which at least some insight is maintained.

- **"Bizarre" delusions.** It is not clear that the bizarre–nonbizarre distinction has much reliability or predictive validity. Some delusions (e.g., somatic delusions, delusions of jealousy) are inherently more plausible than others. Consider, for instance, "I know I have cancer no matter what the tests say" versus "My actions are controlled by a microchip implanted in my brain by aliens before I was born." But at the boundaries, one person's "plausible" is another's "bizarre."

- **Hallucinations.** These are usually absent in Delusional Disorder, but there is one exception: Some people are delusionally concerned about being offensive to others and may have olfactory hallucinations of smelling bad.

- **Criminal responsibility.** The boundary between Delusional Disorder and ideology is particularly difficult in forensic determinations. For instance, was the Unabomber suffering from Delusional Disorder, or was he making a political statement? Should he be confined to prison or to a psychiatric hospital?

■ 297.3 SHARED PSYCHOTIC DISORDER (FOLIE À DEUX)

Note to readers: DSM-5 eliminated this diagnosis for no apparent reason. Cases do occasionally occur, and the diagnosis has obvious treatment significance.

Screening Question

"Do you share beliefs with a loved one that others find strange?"

Diagnostic Prototype

A dominant person forces his delusion on a submissive person who would not otherwise be psychotic. This probably happens a lot more in the movies than in real life, but I have personally seen four cases over the years, and from time to time a clear case of "folie à cult" hits the headlines. We might even say that Hitler created a "folie à country."

The problem starts with a convincing, charismatic individual who succeeds in selling her delusion—usually one or another version of "It's us against the world." On the clinical level, the duo is usually mother–daughter or husband–wife; the delusional one is extremely forceful and dominant, and the gullible partner is weak, suggestible, and submissive. Doing separate interviews can tip you off that each differs greatly in the certainty of belief. Separation and debriefing can result in dissolution of what was probably not a true delusion in the passive partner.

Diagnostic Tip

- As noted above, DSM-5 has dropped this category; it is now collapsed within Delusional Disorder. Although Shared Psychotic Disorder is rare, it is occasionally seen in clinical practice and needs to be distinguished from simple delusions that do not arise as part of a relationship with a dominant psychotic individual. So when it seems appropriate, feel comfortable making the diagnosis and using the official ICD-9-CM code for it.

■ 298.8 BRIEF PSYCHOTIC DISORDER

Screening Question

"Have you had strange experiences lately?"

Diagnostic Prototype

A previously well-functioning person encounters a stress and flips out for a short period of time—usually under a week, sometimes as long as a month—and then returns to the previous level of functioning. Common environmental precipitants include moving away from home to college, traveling to a foreign country, starting or ending a love relationship, entering prison or the military, or being the victim of a traumatic episode. The patient may have delusions or hallucinations (or both), feels spacey and confused, and may be extremely agitated and impulsive.

Differential Diagnosis: Rule These Disorders Out

- **Schizophrenia.** The symptoms are the same, but their duration is longer than 6 months.
- **Schizophreniform Disorder.** The symptoms are the same, but their duration is longer—between 1 and 6 months.
- **Delirium.** Check the person for level of consciousness, orientation, and cognitive functioning.
- **Malingering.** The person may acquire some gain or off-load responsibility.

See the differential diagnosis for Schizophrenia (above) for additional rule-outs.

Diagnostic Tips

- **Frequency.** Brief Psychotic Disorder is considered rare, but this is probably because of underreporting.
- **Differential diagnoses.** Always think first of substance use in the young; of medical illness or medication side effects in the old; and of

Bipolar or Depressive Disorders at any age. Get a drug screen and check out all medications.

- **Severity.** Just because it is short doesn't mean that Brief Psychotic Disorder is mild or risk-free. A patient unaccustomed to psychosis can have terrible judgment and be particularly agitated and impulsive. Brief hospitalization is usually necessary.

- **Traumatic injury or postpartum onset.** Think of medical causes before assuming that the Brief Psychosis is the result of the psychological stress.

- **Culture.** Brief episodes of markedly aberrant behavior occur under different names and with different manifestations in many cultures around the world. It is not clear whether this is better considered Brief Psychotic Disorder or a culturally sanctioned release of otherwise prohibited feelings or social tensions.

- **Malingering.** Consider whether the symptoms are overdone, and whether being psychotic will relieve legal or other responsibility or remove the person from a feared situation.

■ SUBSTANCE-INDUCED PSYCHOTIC DISORDER

291.5   If Alcohol-Induced Delusions

291.3   If Alcohol-Induced Hallucinations

**292.11   If Delusions Are Induced by Any Other Substance
(Indicate Substance)**

**292.12   If Hallucinations Are Induced by Any Other
Substance (Indicate Substance)**

Screening Question

"Do you have strange experiences when you are under the influence of drugs or alcohol?"

Diagnostic Prototype

Whenever you see a young person with psychotic symptoms, the first reflex should be to consider the role of substances, especially if the leading symptoms are hallucinations. Since the patient is likely to be a reluctant informant, laboratory testing for substance use is highly recommended. Transient psychotic symptoms occur as a routine part of intoxication with many drugs, and less frequently with withdrawal. There is no need to use this diagnosis if the symptoms don't exceed what is expectable for that drug and don't require separate treatment. Many medicines and toxins can also cause psychotic symptoms and should be considered in the differential diagnosis.

Differential Diagnosis: Rule This Condition Out

- **Substance-Induced Delirium.** The person also has clouded consciousness, confusion, and disorientation.

■ 293.XX PSYCHOTIC DISORDER DUE TO ANOTHER MEDICAL CONDITION (INDICATE THE MEDICAL CONDITION)

.81 With Delusions
.82 With Hallucinations

Screening Question

"Have you had strange experiences when you're ill?"

Diagnostic Prototype

This diagnosis should be the first thought in anyone who has late onset of psychotic symptoms, especially hallucinations. Do a thorough medical and neurological search to uncover the possible etiological factors. Psychotic Disorder Due to Another Medical Condition is distinguished from Delirium Due to Another Medical Condition by the absence of clouded consciousness, confusion, and disorientation.

■ 293.89 CATATONIC DISORDER DUE TO ANOTHER MEDICAL CONDITION (INDICATE THE MEDICAL CONDITION)

Diagnostic Prototype

The term "catatonia" describes bizarre motor behavior. The most classic symptom is "waxy flexibility"—the assuming and holding of unusual and uncomfortable postures for what would seem to be impossibly long periods of time. Sometimes the patient will assume any new position molded by the evaluator and proceed to maintain it. Or there may be extreme negativism and refusal to move appropriately. Patients may also remain completely immobile and mute, again for extended durations; this is sometimes associated with the delusional belief that any movement or speech may have catastrophic consequences. Rarely, there is the involuntary copying of other people's movements or repetitions of their words. Rarely, there may also be catatonic excitement—random, purposeless, and heedless motion that can result in self-harm, harm to others, or collapse from exhaustion.

Differential Diagnosis: Rule These Conditions Out

- **Bipolar I Disorder.** The person is experiencing a Manic Episode.
- **Neuroleptic-Induced Movement Disorder.**
- **Schizophrenia** (or any other Psychotic Disorder discussed in this chapter).

Diagnostic Tips

- **Decreasing prevalence.** For unclear reasons, catatonia is much less frequent in psychiatric patients than once was the case.
- **Bipolar I Disorder in young patients.** Because there used to be a Catatonic Type of Schizophrenia, many people associate the two and don't realize that catatonia in young patients is now encountered more frequently as a symptom of mania.
- **Medical illness or medication side effects.** Consider medical (especially neurological) illness or the effects of medication whenever there is a first onset in elderly patients.

■ 298.9 UNSPECIFIED PSYCHOTIC DISORDER

Use the Unspecified code when you have determined that there is a Psychotic Disorder, but there is not enough information to distinguish which one fits best. Often it takes the passage of time and several visits to determine the possible impact of substances or medical illness. This category would also be used for presentations of psychosis that don't resemble any of the specific categories described above.

CAUTION: Attenuated Psychosis Syndrome

Attenuated Psychosis Syndrome is listed in Section 3 of DSM-5 as a proposed diagnosis requiring further research. For several reasons, I recommend that it not be considered or coded under Unspecified Psychotic Disorder:

1. The false-positive rate for this proposed diagnosis is unacceptably high—65% in expert clinics and over 90% in more general practice.
2. These individuals do not have psychotic symptoms, making it inappropriate to include them within a section of DSM devoted to psychosis.
3. There is no treatment of proven effectiveness, making this diagnosis moot.
4. Using the diagnosis risks the possibility that it will be inappropriately treated with antipsychotic medication that may cause extremely harmful side effects.
5. The diagnosis is stigmatizing, usually inaccurate, and can cause needless worry and reduced expectations.
6. There are insufficient data on the most appropriate way of defining Attenuated Psychosis Syndrome. This is a diagnosis suitable only for research, not for clinical practice.

CHAPTER 9

■ Substance-Related Disorders and Behavioral Addictions

IN THIS CHAPTER:

- ■ CAUTION: Substance Abuse and Substance Dependence
- ■ Substance Dependence
- ■ Substance Abuse
- ■ Substance Intoxication
- ■ Substance Withdrawal
- ■ Substance-Induced Mental Disorders
- ■ CAUTION: Pathological Gambling and Other Behavioral Addictions

---

CAUTION:
Substance Abuse and Substance Dependence

DSM-5 collapses the previously separate categories of Substance Abuse and Substance Dependence into one—Substance Use Disorder. Persons with DSM-IV Substance Abuse have thus been relabeled in a way that includes them in the very same category with people who have end-stage addictions.

DSM-5 drew its rationale for combining Substance Dependence and Substance Abuse from a statistical analysis suggesting that there is no sharp boundary between them. This is an unconvincing argument even on research grounds, and it makes absolutely no sense conceptually or clinically. None of the DSM-5 mental disorders has a clear boundary with its near neighbor. We split disorders apart whenever this saves useful information that would be lost if they were lumped together. There is no obvious benefit in joining Substance Dependence and Substance Abuse, and there are three very substantial disadvantages:

1. **Stigma.** It is unfair and damaging to pin the label "addict" on someone whose substance problems are intermittent, may be temporary, and are often very influenced by contextual and developmental factors. Take the example of a college kid in a hard-drinking fraternity who binges on weekends, gets into one fight, and has one arrest for driving while intoxicated. He is obviously already in serious trouble (and flirting with much worse) and needs immediate help. But what is gained by calling him an "addict" and possibly jeopardizing his future marital opportunities, job prospects, licensing, insurance eligibility, and legal status? Most persons with Substance Abuse as defined by DSM-IV are in a passing phase and never become "addicted" in any meaningful sense of that word. The term "addiction" has never (in its entire history of often very loose usage) been used this loosely.

2. **Lost information.** Combining Substance Abuse and Dependence loses much valuable distinguishing information. There is a world of difference in behavior, treatment needs, and prognosis between someone with well-established Substance Dependence and someone with a new and probably temporary Substance Abuse problem. The label Substance Dependence clues the clinician that abstinence may trigger severe physical or psychological withdrawal, requiring a special intensity of medical and rehabilitation response. The intervention for Substance Abuse will be more directed to the harmful consequences of binges, ways to avoid them, and the substitution of other less dangerous recreational activities. There is also a considerable difference in prognosis. While some go on from an early history of Substance Abuse to later Substance Dependence, most do not and are much more likely to have an early and permanent remission.

3. **Wrong message.** The message to the college student in the example above that he is already among the "addicted" has these unfortunate connotations: The substance has already gained a central role in his life; it will be terribly difficult to give up because of psychological and/or physical dependence and painful withdrawal symptoms; all this is somehow biological, fated in the genes, and outside his control or ability to change; and he has a reduced amount of personal responsibility for substance use and its consequences. Being "addicted" can become a self-fulfilling prophecy and a great excuse for not meeting responsibilities to self, family, school, and the legal system.

For all these reasons, I recommend continuing the ICD-approved distinction between Substance Dependence and Substance Abuse and using the different ICD-9-CM codes that are provided for them.

■ SUBSTANCE DEPENDENCE

303.9 Alcohol Dependence

304.40 Amphetamine Dependence

304.30 Cannabis Dependence

304.20 Cocaine Dependence

304.30 Hallucinogen Dependence

304.60 Inhalant Dependence

304.00 Opioid Dependence

304.60 Phencyclidine Dependence

304.10 Sedative, Hypnotic, or Anxiolytic Dependence

305.1 Tobacco Dependence

304.80 Polysubstance Dependence

304.90 Other (or Unknown) Substance Dependence (Indicate Substance If Known)

Screening Question

"Has anyone ever suggested that you have an alcohol or drug problem?"

Diagnostic Prototype

Tolerance, withdrawal, and compulsive use are the three hallmarks of Substance Dependence. The person needs more and more of the substance to get the same effect ("tolerance"), and trying to stop brings on painful physical and psychological symptoms ("withdrawal").

Rather than enjoying the drug, he now needs it. He no longer controls the substance; the substance controls him, and he feels compelled to use even though it is ruining his life ("compulsive use"). He may desperately want to stop but can't; a strong craving keeps bringing him back for more.

Differential Diagnosis: Rule These Conditions Out

- **Recreational use.** Even heavy substance use that doesn't cause clinically significant impairment or distress.
- **Substance Abuse.** The person gets into significant trouble because of using the substance, but there is no tolerance, withdrawal, or pattern of compulsive use.

Diagnostic Tips

- **Informants.** People with Substance Dependence are uniquely poor judges (and even worse reporters) of their degree of substance use and of the severity of its impact on their lives. Always bring in outside informants to get a more complete and accurate picture.

- **Laboratory testing.** This is often eye-opening. I can't count how many times I have been fooled by the sincerest claims of abstinence.

- **Patterns.** Some drugs cause physiological dependence and compulsive use (e.g., alcohol, cocaine, stimulants, opioids, and sedatives). Other drugs cause only compulsive use (e.g., cannabis, hallucinogens, inhalants, PCP).

- **Compulsive use.** This is evidenced by the person's centering his entire life around substance use, and also being unable to quit despite powerful health, family, or work motivations to do so.

- **Recreational use.** As indicated above, this doesn't count as a mental disorder unless there is clinically significant impairment or distress.

- **Recreational use versus compulsive use.** This difficult distinction depends on judging whether the person's substance use is understandable, given the pleasure–cost ratio. Do the harmful consequences overwhelm the pleasure? The judgment is influenced by varying individual, family, cultural, and clinical interpretations of what is reasonable recreational fun versus what crosses the threshold of clinically significant distress and impairment.

- **Caffeine.** Compulsive caffeine use is so common and for most people harmless that it is almost normative and is not considered an addiction.

- **Remission under special conditions.** It is helpful to use the DSM-IV specifiers for external factors that may play a necessary role in maintaining remission—most commonly On Agonist Therapy (e.g., methadone) or In A Controlled Environment (e.g., prison).

- **Cultural factors.** Cultures vary widely in their attitudes to drinking (Mediterranean wine drinking as a way of life vs. Islamic prohibitions of it as the path of sin). A wine-loving Frenchman may be physiologically hooked, but may not qualify for a diagnosis of Substance Dependence because he experiences no clinically significant distress or impairment.

- **Substance Dependence as an essential part of every evaluation.** Substance Dependence is a frequent hidden factor in the presentation of virtually every psychiatric disorder. You usually won't find out about it unless you ask, and even then it is often undisclosed, especially during the early evaluation period. Think about the possible role of substance use and Substance Dependence in every single patient you see.

■ SUBSTANCE ABUSE

305.00 Alcohol Abuse

305.70 Amphetamine Abuse

305.20 Cannabis Abuse

305.60 Cocaine Abuse

305.30 Hallucinogen Abuse

305.90 Inhalant Abuse

305.50 Opioid Abuse

305.90 Phencyclidine Abuse

305.40 Sedative, Hypnotic, or Anxiolytic Abuse

305.90 Other (or Unknown) Substance Abuse (Indicate Substance If Known)

Screening Question

"Have you gotten into trouble because of alcohol or drugs?"

Diagnostic Prototype

Substance Abuse is defined by serious adverse consequences occurring in the absence of tolerance, withdrawal, or compulsive use. The typical person with Substance Abuse gets into recurrent but intermittent (often weekend) trouble as a consequence of episodic binges. There are periods when he seems able to take or leave the substance, use it in a controlled way, or abstain from it altogether. Then comes a bender with a bad outcome, another peaceful period, then another destructive bender, and so on. The person doesn't learn from the repeated painful experience that a couple of drinks (or snorts or pills or joints) can lead to a binge, and that a binge can, and often does, have serious (and sometimes even catastrophic) consequences: arrests for driving while intoxicated and/or car accidents;

bar fights; getting fired for drinking or using on the job; marital discord; neglect of parental responsibility; spending excessively; and sometimes even committing crimes.

Differential Diagnosis: Rule These Conditions Out

- **Recreational use.** The person doesn't get into trouble because of substance use, and there is no clinically significant distress or impairment.
- **Substance Dependence.** Tolerance, withdrawal, and/or a pattern of compulsive use are present.

Diagnostic Tips

- **Informants.** As noted in regard to Substance Dependence, people are poor judges and poor reporters of their substance use and the problems it causes. Bring in outside informants whenever possible.
- **Laboratory testing.** Again, this provides another source of valuable information.
- **Course.** For some, Substance Abuse is a stable pattern of unstable life, but most people either outgrow it or go on to Substance Dependence. The threshold between the two is crossed when the periodic bingeing turns into continuous use and the motivation switches from pleasurable recreation to needing the substance on a regular basis just to get by.
- **Recreational binges.** Substance Abuse must be distinguished from run-of-the-mill bingeing. Binges do not qualify as a mental disorder unless they are repetitive and cause clinically significant distress or impairment.
- **Family history of Substance Dependence.** Family history is a risk factor that the Substance Abuse will eventually evolve into Substance Dependence.
- **Other risk factors.** These include an early onset, heavy and frequent use, or an inherited high tolerance.
- **Lethality.** Substance Abuse can be one of the most dangerous disorders in psychiatry. It takes only one incident of driving while intoxicated to result in multiple deaths by car accident.
- **Prevention.** Substance Abuse is the strongest indication in psychiatry for early identification and active intervention.

■ SUBSTANCE INTOXICATION

303.00 Alcohol Intoxication

292.89 Intoxication With Any Other Substance (Indicate Substance)

292.89 Other (or Unknown) Substance Intoxication (Indicate Substance If Known)

Screening Question

"Do you ever get into trouble when you get drunk or high on drugs?"

Diagnostic Prototype

Substance Intoxication is a set of symptoms and behaviors that occurs shortly after taking a substance. It usually lasts only a short time, after which the person returns to the previous state. Each substance has a characteristic pattern of intoxication that accounts for its widespread recreational popularity.

The common problems resulting from intoxication are cognitive impairment, perceptual disturbances, reduced or increased arousal, poor judgment, emotional lability, impulsivity, agitation, sleep disturbance, disinhibition of angry and sexual impulses, and reckless behavior.

Differential Diagnosis: Rule This Condition Out

• **Recreational use.** Do not diagnose Substance Intoxication to describe expectable recreational responses or cognitive impairments that do not cause clinically significant distress or behavioral impairment.

■ SUBSTANCE WITHDRAWAL

291.81 Alcohol Withdrawal

292.0 Withdrawal from Any Other Substance (Indicate Substance)

292.0 Other (or Unknown) Substance Withdrawal (Indicate Substance If Known)

Screening Question

"Do you ever get troubling symptoms when you try to stop drinking or using a drug?"

Diagnostic Prototype

Withdrawal from a substance often produces a set of psychological and physical symptoms representing a rebound from the substance's intoxicating effects. As with Substance Intoxication, no diagnosis of Substance Withdrawal as a mental disorder is needed if the withdrawal syndrome is not causing clinically significant distress or behavioral impairment. The symptoms of withdrawal generally persist for days to weeks, depending on the substance and the pattern and duration of its prior use.

Differential Diagnosis: Rule This Condition Out

- **Uncomplicated withdrawal from recreational use.** Again, no diagnosis of a mental disorder is needed if the withdrawal syndrome is not causing clinically significant distress or behavioral impairment.

■ SUBSTANCE-INDUCED MENTAL DISORDERS

Screening Question

"Tell me about your use of alcohol and drugs."

Diagnostic Prototype

Substance use can cause or amplify virtually all of the psychiatric disorders (Psychotic Disorders, Bipolar or Depressive Disorders, Anxiety Disorders, OCD, Sexual Dysfunctions, and more).

Substances are widely used, and their use is often underreported. They are a hidden source of a significant proportion of all the psychiatric problems that need to be diagnosed. It is always crucial to inquire about substance use and to consider its role in the presentation.

Specific Substance-Induced Disorders are included in the other chapters in this book with the non-substance-related presentations that each most closely mimics. This is meant to provide convenience in the differential diagnosis.

Diagnostic Tips

- **The importance of substance use.** As emphasized above, use of substances can cause or amplify virtually all of the psychiatric disorders; it is widespread; and it often goes unreported or underreported. It is always crucial to inquire about substance use and consider its possible role in every psychiatric presentation.
- **Confusion in the clinical picture.** Any use of substances in the context of mental disorder makes diagnosis more difficult and treatment less likely to be effective.
- **Establishing cause and effect.** It is often unclear whether (1) the substance use is causing the psychiatric problem; (2) it is a means of secondary self-medication; or (3) the substance use and the mental disorder are independent. Evaluate the chronology of onsets, the prominence of the substance use in the clinical picture, and whether the psychiatric symptoms are the ones characteristically caused by that specific substance.
- **Getting the person off the substance.** The best tool in determining the diagnosis is also the best tool in treating the patient—that is, getting the person off the substance and seeing what happens. Of course, this is often far easier said than done.
- **Relation to Substance Intoxication and Withdrawal.** The diagnoses of Substance Intoxication and Substance Withdrawal are superseded whenever either causes a more specific, severe, and persistent Substance-Induced Mental Disorder. But don't diagnose a Substance-Induced Mental Disorder if the symptoms are not particularly persistent or more severe than would be expected from routine intoxication or withdrawal.

CAUTION: Pathological Gambling and Other Behavioral Addictions

DSM-5's section on Substance-Related and Addictive Disorders includes Pathological Gambling and introduces the new and problematic concept of Behavioral Addictions. (For a fuller discussion of Pathological Gambling, see Chapter 12.) Fortunately, none of the other Behavioral Addictions originally suggested for DSM-5 has gained official status. But the risk remains that "addictions" to video games, sex, shopping, exercise, working, and so on will become increasingly popular and loosely applied as mental disorders.

The Rationale for Behavioral Addictions

The rationale for Behavioral Addictions is that compulsive behaviors and compulsive substance use create similar subjective experiences, follow the same clinical pattern, may derive from the same neural network, and respond to similar treatments. The notion underlying the "addiction" concept is that the substance use (or behavior) originally intended for pleasurable recreation is now compulsively driven. Although the act is no longer the source of much pleasure, it has become so deeply ingrained that the person continues to perform it in a repetitive fashion, despite great and mounting negative consequences. Subjectively, the person feels an escalating loss of control over the substance or the act, and instead comes to feel increasingly controlled by it.

The Problem: Compulsion versus Recreational Pleasure

There is, however, a fundamental problem with the idea of Behavioral Addictions. Repetitive (even if quite costly) pleasure seeking is a ubiquitous part of human nature, whereas compulsive behavior that is not rewarding is rare. But it is extremely difficult to tell the two apart. Behavioral Addictions can quickly be expanded from narrowly intended and (perhaps occasionally) appropriate usage to become a popular and much misused label for anything that people do for fun, but causes them trouble.

With the new category of Behavioral Addictions, potentially millions of new "patients" can be created by fiat. The label may medicalize all manner of pleasure-seeking behaviors and give people a "sick role" excuse for irresponsibly pursuing them to excess.

CHAPTER 10
■ Neurocognitive Disorders

■ DELIRIUM

293.0 Delirium Due to Another Medical Condition (Indicate the Medical Condition)

Name each specific diagnosis according to the particular medical condition (e.g., Delirium Due to HIV Encephalitis).

Substance-Induced Delirium

291.0   If Alcohol-Induced
292.81 If Induced by Any Other Substance (Indicate Substance)
780.09 Unspecified Delirium

Screening Questions for Any Delirium

To the informant: "Is your husband confused and acting strangely?"

To the patient: "Who is that lady sitting next to you? What kind of place is this? Why did she bring you here? What season of the year is this? What year? What time of day? What did you have for breakfast? Subtract 3 from 100, and then keep subtracting 3 from the new number. Spell 'world' backward."

Diagnostic Prototype for Any Delirium

Delirium often signals an urgent and dangerous medical emergency that requires immediate diagnosis and active intervention. The onset is usually sudden and the course short. The patient either (1) gets better, (2) suffers permanent brain damage, or (3) dies. Death can result from the underlying medical illness or from the fatal consequences of the patient's impulsive and erratic behavior.

Delirium seriously impairs every aspect of attention, thinking, feeling, and behaving. The manifestations are protean and fluctuate in severity, sometimes from minute to minute. Consciousness is clouded; attention is spotty; and the patient is distractible, confused, and unable to focus. Reality testing is tenuous, and the person floats in and out of contact with the environment—often being disoriented to time and place, and sometimes even to person. All cognitive functions are impaired, and judgment is poor to nonexistent. The person is likely to have perceptual distortions (especially visual illusions or hallucinations) and may have severe misinterpretations of reality or even frank delusions. Emotions are labile, intense, disinhibited, and often terrifying. There can be too much or too little sleep and/or a reversal of the usual sleep–wake cycle. Things are bad during the day and usually much worse at night. Agitation is often intense, and the patient may become verbally aggressive and/or physically violent. Often Delirium is unmistakable, but sometimes it can be all too easy to miss, especially in a quiet and obtunded patient whose confusion is unobtrusive.

Differential Diagnosis: Rule These Conditions Out for Any Delirium

- **Major Neurocognitive Disorder (Dementia).** Cognitive problems are long-term, stable, and without an acute clouding of consciousness.
- **Dementia with superimposed Delirium.** The two frequently occur together.
- **Delirium due to multiple etiologies.** For example, a person with Substance Abuse who experiences head trauma, or someone with severe congestive heart failure who is also taking eight medicines, may develop Delirium.
- **Substance Intoxication or Withdrawal.** The symptoms are no more than is usual for that substance.
- **A primary Psychotic Disorder.** The person is more likely to have auditory than visual hallucinations.
- **A primary Bipolar, Depressive, or Anxiety Disorder.** Consider when panic, anxiety, agitation, or depression are prominent without change in consciousness or confusion or visual hallucinations.
- **Acute Stress Disorder or PTSD.** The confusion and agitation result from psychological trauma, not neurological compromise.
- **Malingering.** Consider this when faking confusion and disorientation might confer some gain.

Diagnostic Tips for Any Delirium

- **Delirium is a medical emergency.** Never forget that untreated Delirium is brain-damaging and life-threatening. Think and act fast.

- **The need for consultation.** And don't think and act alone. Get a medical consultation as soon as possible.

- **The need for a high index of suspicion.** Don't be fooled into thinking that symptoms arise from a primary mental disorder when there is an acute brain insult to identify and treat. Once Delirium is in the differential diagnosis, the assessment of mental status must be accompanied by an urgent exploration to determine and treat possible medical causes before more damage is done to the vulnerable brain.

- **Medication overdosing.** Elderly patients are often taking multiple drugs that are cleared less well by their aging kidneys and livers. Medication interactions and overdose are major causes of Delirium in the elderly and should be first on any list of usual suspects.

- **Delirium versus a primary Psychotic, Bipolar, or Depressive Disorder.** Whenever there are visual hallucinations, think Delirium and act fast; these are much less common in Psychotic, Bipolar, and Depressive Disorders. Delirium also typically has a much, much later age of initial onset.

- **Delirium versus Acute Stress Disorder.** Delirium can be missed after a traumatic event (e.g., a car accident) if the terror, confusion, agitation, startle, and autonomic arousal are mislabeled as PTSD symptoms and the visual hallucinations are mislabeled as flashbacks.

- **"Sundowning."** Symptoms worsen at night with reduced orienting cues, and there are sleep–wake reversals. To prevent sundowning, try a night light, personal attention, and orientation hints.

- **Stress, environmental changes, a minor illness, pain, or overmedication.** All these can trigger Delirium in people who have Dementia.

- **Structuring the environment.** Pictures, calendars, routines, familiar objects, and familiar people can all help to orient and reduce confusion. Again, a night light can help as well.

- **EEG findings.** Generalized slowing on EEG can help confirm Delirium in doubtful cases.

- **The quiet patient.** The patient with agitated Delirium who causes trouble is likely to get adequate attention. Don't miss the quiet, obtunded patient who doesn't make a fuss.

■ MAJOR NEUROCOGNITIVE DISORDER (DEMENTIA)

In DSM-5, the term Dementia has been replaced by Major and Minor Neurocognitive Disorders. See the Caution box at the end of this chapter for my serious reservations about Minor Neurocognitive Disorder. And for simplicity's sake, I will continue to use Dementia in the diagnoses listed below and in this section's discussions.

294.xx Dementia Due to Alzheimer's Disease
  .10 With Behavioral Disturbance
  .11 Without Behavioral Disturbance
290.xx Vascular Dementia
  .40 Uncomplicated
  .41 With Delirium
  .42 With Delusions
  .43 With Depressed Mood
294.xx Dementia Due to Traumatic Brain Injury
  .10 With Behavioral Disturbance
  .11 Without Behavioral Disturbance
294.xx Dementia Due to Parkinson's Disease
  .10 With Behavioral Disturbance
  .11 Without Behavioral Disturbance
294.xx Dementia Due to Lewy Body Disease
  .10 With Behavioral Disturbance
  .11 Without Behavioral Disturbance
294.xx Dementia Due to HIV Infection
  .10 With Behavioral Disturbance
  .11 Without Behavioral Disturbance
294.xx Dementia Due to Frontotemporal Lobar Degeneration
  .10 With Behavioral Disturbance
  .11 Without Behavioral Disturbance

294.xx **Dementia Due to Huntington's Disease**
.10 **With Behavioral Disturbance**
.11 **Without Behavioral Disturbance**
294.xx **Dementia Due to Prion Disease**
.10 **With Behavioral Disturbance**
.11 **Without Behavioral Disturbance**

Substance-Induced Persisting Dementia

291.2 **If Alcohol-Induced**
292.82 **If Induced by Any Other Substance (Indicate Substance)**

Screening Question for Any Dementia

"Have you [or a loved one] had a big decline in memory?"

Diagnostic Prototype for Any Dementia

"Gentlemen, you see before you the wreck of what once was a pretty good man." These were the unforgettable words of the first patient I ever saw in medical school. He was a physician in the middle stages of Dementia who could describe his cognitive decline with haunting clinical precision. It had begun gradually with mild memory impairment that by now was quite dense. He could still recall obscure details from his childhood and accurately describe many medical illnesses, but he could not remember what he had eaten for breakfast or what he had just said (and might repeat the same thought over and over again 15 times within an hour). He had once conducted an efficient and well-organized medical practice, but now he could not handle a checkbook, figure out change, make or keep an appointment, or decide what to order from a menu. Lately he had wandered away from home several times and could not find his way back without the help of neighbors or the police. People with more severe Dementia will forget who family members are; will develop severe difficulties with language and retrieving the names of things; will be befuddled by seemingly simple activities like dressing or brushing teeth; and will have trouble identifying and figuring out the purpose of everyday objects (e.g., what the difference between a dime and a dollar is, or how to use a hair dryer). There may be disinhibition of aggressive and/or sexual impulses, poor judgment, and impetuous behavior. The savings of a lifetime can be squandered within months. The person is often unaware of the limitations imposed by the illness and may be vulnerable to exploitation.

Differential Diagnosis: Rule These Conditions Out for Any Dementia

- **Age-Related Cognitive Decline.** Symptoms are gradual, are age-appropriate, and do not cause loss of independence or clinically significant distress or impairment. Code this 780.9 (see Chapter 18).
- **Delirium.** Cognitive deficits are acute, and clouding consciousness is prominent.
- **Dementia with superimposed Delirium.** As noted earlier, the two frequently occur together.
- **Intellectual Developmental Disorder.** Onset of cognitive deficits is before age 18.
- **Substance Intoxication or Withdrawal.** Either may make a person seem much more cognitively disabled than he really is.
- **A primary Mood Disorder.** Cognitive deficits are restricted to a Major Depressive Episode.
- **Schizophrenia.** The person has cognitive deficits, but with early onset and a different pattern.
- **Malingering.** There is some obvious gain for the person. One example was the New York City Mafia leader who for many years wandered the streets in his pajamas, talking to himself and acting confused, in order to convince the FBI that he couldn't possibly still be the boss of his crime family.

Diagnostic Tips for Any Dementia

- **Careful, deliberate diagnosis.** Don't assume that Dementia lurks in every unrecalled fact, forgotten face, or irretrievable name. Normal aging includes loss of cognitive skills, and Dementia should be considered only when the decrements go well beyond what is expected and cause significant impairment.

- **Careful medical and neurological evaluation.** Recommend a thorough medical workup to rule out possibly reversible causes of Dementia.

- **Informants.** Part of Dementia is that the patient is often the last to know he has it. Get as much information as possible from the people in the patient's life.

- **Laboratory testing.** Everyone is looking forward to finally having a panel of biological tests for Alzheimer's disease, and such tests will probably be available in a few years. Unfortunately, testing for Alzheimer's won't do much good if we can't treat it effectively, and an effective treatment appears to be a long way off.

- **Dementia as a global illness.** Although the leading symptoms are cognitive, the deficits in brain functioning are pervasive and also profoundly affect emotions and behavior.

- **Dementia versus a primary Bipolar or Depressive Disorder.** Dementia can mimic a Bipolar or Depressive Disorder, and vice versa. The disorders are often hard to distinguish, and errors of diagnosis are made in both directions. Things are even more complicated because Dementia and a Bipolar or Depressive Disorder can occur together. The differential diagnosis requires careful medical and neuropsychological evaluation and close longitudinal monitoring. Always be especially thorough in looking for preventable causes of Dementia whenever there are profound cognitive symptoms accompanying a Bipolar or Depressive Disorder.

- **Practical mental status testing.** Ask questions of direct relevance to the patient's current life, to help determine the impact of the memory impairment on daily functioning. "Do you find yourself losing your car in a parking lot or having trouble finding your way home?" "Do you sometimes forget to turn off the stove?" "Are you having trouble recognizing people you should know?"

- **Safety first.** Assess the risks of possible self-harm (e.g., misusing kitchen appliances, falling in the shower, wandering off, aggressiveness, sexually inappropriate behavior, financial vulnerability, etc.).

- **Driving.** This deserves special mention because people are extremely stubborn about giving up the freedom of the open road and often have especially poor judgment about how badly their driving skills have deteriorated. Emphasize that they can kill not only themselves but others, including small children. Encourage family members to be proactive, to confiscate keys, and to consult the local Department of Motor Vehicles. This is not punitive; it is just common sense.

- **Environmental modifications.** Make the world less complicated; provide auxiliary help; and create a familiar environment with lots of orienting cues.
- **Catastrophic reactions.** Patients with Dementia sometimes have "emotional incontinence"—excessively angry, sad, or fearful reactions that are very far out of proportion to the stress. Don't overreact to their overreactions. They will usually soon get over it and just move on as if nothing has happened.
- **Falling.** Dementia is a risk factor. The environment needs to be as free as possible of potential obstacles.

■ MILD NEUROCOGNITIVE DISORDER

DSM-5 has added a new diagnostic category that it calls Mild Neurocognitive Disorder, but I strongly advise against its use. See the Caution box below.

CAUTION: Mild Neurocognitive Disorder

DSM-5 includes the new diagnostic category of Mild Neurocognitive Disorder to identify people with problems that don't yet, but later may, qualify for a diagnosis of Major Neurocognitive Disorder (Dementia). The definition requires mild impairments in cognitive function that do not yet threaten independence or the performance of activities of daily living. There are many serious problems with using this diagnosis that suggest it is not yet ready for "prime time."

1. **High false-positive rate.** With aging, people naturally begin to lose cognitive skills just as they gradually lose physical skills. There is no bright line separating what should be labeled "illness" from what is the expectable wear and tear of life. This is particularly true, given the vast individual differences in previous baseline functioning, in self-expectations, and in the cognitive challenges that have to be faced. There will be an unacceptably high false-positive rate, surely exceeding 50%.
2. **Fallible clinical criteria.** The DSM-5 definition of Mild Neurocognitive Disorder is based exclusively on extremely fallible and unreliable clinical criteria.
3. **Role of biological tests.** Accurate diagnosis of Mild Neurocognitive Disorder will most certainly require biological tests. And these are now within reach. Within

the next few years, we will have objective laboratory methods to identify the prodrome of Alzheimer's disease. Much remains to be done in standardizing these tests, determining their appropriate set points and patterns of results, and negotiating the difficult transition from research to general clinical practice, but the goal is within sight. The rapidly advancing science makes obvious how premature it is now to attempt to diagnose Mild Neurocognitive Disorder on the basis of vague and untested clinical criteria. No purpose can be served by rushing ahead with a second-rate clinical method of prodrome diagnosis when more accurate biological testing will so soon be available.

4. **Creation of needless worries and stigma without any benefit.** There is currently no effective treatment for Mild Neurocognitive Disorder, and none is obvious on the near horizon. The diagnosis does no real good even for people who are accurately diagnosed. Why scare people with an ominous diagnosis when it is so likely to be inaccurate and panic-producing, and when it provides no useful call to action?

5. **An idea not ready for clinical prime time.** Mild Neurocognitive Disorder is a research idea that is far out of touch with current clinical reality and is simply not ready for general use.

I recommend against the current use of the diagnosis Mild Neurocognitive Disorder until it can be established by laboratory testing. Diagnosis based on vague clinical criteria is risky, untested, irrelevant, and inaccurate, and will cause far more harm than good. "First, do no harm."

■ 294.8 UNSPECIFIED NEUROCOGNITIVE DISORDER

Unspecified Neurocognitive Disorder is a useful placeholder in the not-uncommon situation of uncertainty whether cognitive deficits are due to Delirium, Dementia, or a combination of both.

CHAPTER 11
■ Personality Disorders

IN THIS CHAPTER:

- Borderline Personality Disorder
- Antisocial Personality Disorder
- Narcissistic Personality Disorder
- Histrionic Personality Disorder
- Obsessive–Compulsive Personality Disorder
- Avoidant Personality Disorder
- Dependent Personality Disorder
- Paranoid Personality Disorder
- Schizoid Personality Disorder
- Schizotypal Personality Disorder
- Personality Change Due to Another Medical Condition (Indicate the Medical Condition)
- Unspecified Personality Disorder
- CAUTION: Avoiding Forensic Use of Unspecified Personality Disorder
- CAUTION: Personality Dimensions in DSM-5's Section 3

Screening Question for Any Personality Disorder

"Do you have a style of doing things and relating to people that gets you into the same kind of mess over and over again?"

Diagnostic Prototype for Any Personality Disorder

In Shakespeare's *Julius Caesar*, Cassius says, "The fault, dear Brutus, is not in our stars, but in ourselves. . . ." Our characters strongly influence our fate. How we see the world and respond to it very much determines how the world sees and responds to us. "Personality" is an enduring pattern of thinking, feeling, interacting, and behaving that is who we are; it provides the texture of our relations with other people. Personality Disorders cause vicious cycles of negative expectation and self-fulfilling prophecies. Normal personality traits become Personality Disorders when they are inflexible and make people unable to adapt to the needs of the moment. The diagnosis of a Personality Disorder is made only if the resulting problems cause clinically significant distress or impairment.

Specific Diagnostic Prototypes for Each Personality Disorder

301.83 Borderline Personality Disorder

The patients have intense and frustrating relationships, filled with high hopes that degenerate into fierce fights and terrible disappointments. Terrified of abandonment, they drive people away with unrealistic demands, unrelenting anger, and self-fulfilling expectations that they will be rejected. Real or imagined losses may lead to suicide attempts and/or self-mutilation, usually with a razor or cigarette. They have repeated destructive relationships, as well as an unsure sense of self, and may display impulsive sexual and aggressive behaviors. The lifetime suicide rate is high (10%), but those who survive often experience improvement and mellowing out with middle age.

301.7 Antisocial Personality Disorder

Bad apples from early on, these people displayed early symptoms of Conduct Disorder; went through a juvenile delinquent stage; and have grown up into selfish, manipulative, and ruthless adults whose interest in other people extends only so far as they can extract things from them. Their brimming charm disguises cold hearts and calculating souls. They lie, cheat, and manipulate without empathy or remorse for the considerable harm they do to others. They are reckless, impulsive, and likely to run afoul of the law. Antisocial Personality Disorder is particularly common among criminals and is a predictor of violence and suicide. Fortunately, like Borderline Personality Disorder, Antisocial Personality Disorder often improves with maturation into middle age.

301.81 Narcissistic Personality Disorder

The patients are the center of their worlds—special in every way, show-offs and name droppers, legends in their own minds. Their sense of self-importance and entitlement crowds out any worries about the needs, troubles, or feelings of others. They are haughty, high-handed, and superior, and expect others to show deference and admiration. Frequent disappointments follow when they and the world fail to live up to impossibly unrealistic expectations.

301.50 Histrionic Personality Disorder

She is a Blanche DuBois—always the exhibitionistic belle of the ball, using charm, physical appeal, and flirty seductiveness to hold center stage. Her relationships and emotions are intense, but shallow and always shifting.

He commands attention by bragging about insider stock tips or prowess on the tennis court. His interests and attitudes are easily influenced by other people or by the role he is currently playing. He comes on strong and is quickly intimate in relationships, but he wears thin quickly and feels unappreciated.

301.4 Obsessive–Compulsive Personality Disorder

These individuals are perfectionists and inflexible control freaks who have to get every last detail just right. Delegating to others is impossible because the others can never be trusted to be nearly careful enough. Life is controlled by rules, schedules, and rigid routines. Their scrupulous attention to work robs them of spontaneity, relaxation, or deep relationships. They are stingy with money, emotions, and affection, and they make it clear that it always has to be "their way or the highway."

301.82 Avoidant Personality Disorder

These people are frightened, socially awkward, and extremely sensitive to criticism or rejection. Any new social contact engenders the terror of possible humiliation and a shrinking away from possible embarrassment. It is far simpler to say a quick "no" to every new work or social relationship that might threaten the safety of their cocoon. In contrast to those with Schizoid Personality Disorder, they crave relationships and usually have some old friends with whom they feel safe and close enough to relax.

301.6 Dependent Personality Disorder

These are people who feel stupid and weak—unable to care for themselves, make their own decisions, or be alone. Their neediness makes them submissive and subservient, willing to put other people's needs and views ahead of their own. They will do whatever it takes to get someone to care for and nurture them, give them affection, and provide their life with direction.

301.0 Paranoid Personality Disorder

The world is a dangerous place, and people are never to be trusted—even (maybe especially) those who are closest. They have to keep alert at all times to make sure that someone is not taking advantage of them, making fun of them, or plotting against them. They never share their thoughts or feelings because these will surely be used against them. They never forget a slight, give up a grudge, or pass up a chance to collect an injustice.

301.20 Schizoid Personality Disorder

These individuals basically just want to be left alone. Having contact with others is empty, without pleasure, emotion, comfort, or meaning. They pick the most solitary of occupations, live alone, avoid dating, and have no real friends. Others find them to be "cold fishes"—awkward, distant, and formal in all social contacts.

301.22 Schizotypal Personality Disorder

The patients have disorganized speech, disorganized behavior, and emotional blunting, but without the delusions and hallucinations that would convert the diagnosis to Schizophrenia. There are eccentricities of thought and behavior, weird beliefs, and strange perceptual experiences, but all these consistently fall short of being frankly psychotic. The symptoms and behaviors have an early onset, are part of who the person is, and generally remain stable throughout life.

Note: Many of these individuals are now being diagnosed (or self-diagnose) as having Asperger's Disorder because this has become much more socially acceptable, provides access to a rich Internet support community, and is more likely to open doors to school and other services.

310.1 Personality Change Due to Another Medical Condition (Indicate the Medical Condition)

Personality Disorder always has an early onset and persistent course. If someone's personality seems to change or deteriorate later in life, consider the possibility that a medical or neurological condition (e.g., head trauma, brain tumor) is responsible.

301.9 Unspecified Personality Disorder

Often people display features of two or more of the different personality types described above, but with none of them severe enough by itself to be considered a Personality Disorder. Unspecified Personality Disorder can be used when the combination of characteristics causes clinically significant distress or impairment.

CAUTION: Avoiding Forensic Use of Unspecified Personality Disorder

The diagnosis of Unspecified Personality Disorder is sometimes used inappropriately in "sexually violent predator" hearings. This diagnosis is inherently unreliable and has no place in expert testimony.

Differential Diagnosis: Rule These Conditions Out for Any Personality Disorder

- **Normal personality traits.** There is no clinically significant distress or impairment.
- **Another mental disorder.** The behaviors follow the onset of the other disorder and remit when it gets better.
- **Substance Use Disorders.** The behaviors occur only as a result of Substance Intoxication or Dependence.
- **Personality Change Due to Another Medical Condition.** Examples of such conditions include head trauma and brain tumor.
- **Adjustment Disorder.** Behaviors are a transient response to external stress.

Diagnostic Tips

- **When to assess.** It is not a good idea to evaluate for the presence of a Personality Disorder if the person is in the midst of a Major Depressive Episode, a Manic Episode, or any other major episode of mental disorder. Such an episode will necessarily interfere with (most often worsen) or disguise the person's usual level of personality functioning. For similar reasons, it makes sense to postpone personality evaluation when people are in the midst of a life crisis like divorce, job loss, or bereavement.
- **Whom to evaluate.** It is inherent to Personality Disorders that these individuals are often not very helpful informants about themselves. Someone with Narcissistic Personality Disorder is unlikely to be aware of (much less to own up to) lack of empathy, grandiosity, or exploitative treatment of others. You can't expect an honest self-appraisal from someone with Antisocial Personality Disorder. The more sources of information the better; family members, friends, and records all help to create a fuller and more accurate picture.
- **How to evaluate.** There are standardized, reliable interviewing instruments for evaluating Personality Disorders, but these take far too much time and training for average clinical practice. You will probably have to rely on your clinical intuitions in matching the individual's current behavior to one of the personality prototypes described above. To establish that a Personality Disorder is present, ensure that the age of

onset was early in the person's life; that the features are persistent and continuous; that they are pervasive in every aspect of functioning, not occurring just in response to one person, one stress, or one situation; and that the personality style causes clinically significant distress and/or impairment. This will take time to evaluate, and your impressions may change and deepen as you get to know the patient better.

- **Why to evaluate.** A Personality Disorder is a predictor of course, most effective treatment approach, treatment compliance, treatment response, and risk of suicide.
- **Children and teenagers.** It is usually not a good idea to give people a Personality Disorder diagnosis early in their lives, when behaviors are fluid and unstable. The track record is short; developmental issues render current behavior a poor predictor of the future; and substance use is often dramatically affecting the presentation.
- **Age effects.** People often mellow with age. This is particularly true of those with Borderline and Antisocial Personality Disorders. But aging may bring special problems for people with Narcissistic, Histrionic, and Obsessive–Compulsive Personality Disorders.
- **Late onset.** By definition, there is no late-onset Personality Disorder. If there is a sudden change for the worse in personality functioning, search for the cause. The most likely explanations are the onset of another mental disorder (e.g., depression); the impact of substance use; a neurological problem (head injury, brain tumor); or an overwhelming life stress.
- **Cultural factors.** Different cultures have different prototypes of what is considered to be appropriate personality functioning and what is considered disordered personality. In judging whether someone's personality is deviating from the norm sufficiently for it to be deemed disordered, the standard should be the norm from the patient's own culture, not yours.
- **Observer bias.** We all have our own personalities, and these are likely to influence the way we see and evaluate the personality of others. Self-awareness of one's own personality style is an evaluator's best protection against allowing it to bias judgments on the presence or absence of Personality Disorders in the people being evaluated.

CAUTION:
Personality Dimensions in DSM-5's Section 3

DSM-5 made a courageous attempt to combine the traditional categorical method of Personality Disorder diagnosis with a new and innovative dimensional method. The intention is laudable, but the result was a failure and had to be relegated to DSM-5's Section 3, for diagnoses and other material requiring further study.

Advantages of Dimensional Systems

Dimensional numbers are more accurate than categorical names in describing continuous phenomena (like Personality Disorders, which merge imperceptibly into normality, into other mental disorders, and into one another). The lack of clear boundaries makes a categorical system of personality diagnosis clumsy and inaccurate. Much information is lost when we are forced to classify as white or black something that is an intermediate shade of gray. Dimensional personality diagnosis has long been appealing because numbers are more accurate than names in describing anything (like a Personality Disorder) with unclear boundaries, a continuous distribution, and the ability to be reduced to numerical description. This is precisely why we choose dimensions (not names) to describe IQ, height, and weight, and why we so love computers that crunch numbers in modeling the world.

Advantages of Categorical Systems

People also love naming. Categorical distinctions have the advantage of being more vivid, more familiar, and better able to abstract figure from ground. Categories reflect how most people, and almost all clinicians, think.

The Proposed DSM-5 Hybrid System

Attempting to take advantage of both methods, the DSM-5 Personality and Personality Disorders Work Group created a hybrid model of personality diagnosis that instead managed to combine both methods' worst features. It was a grand idea, but its execution failed. The system included in DSM-5's Section 3 is untested, cumbersome, and impractical—acceptable to no one but the small group of its creators. It serves no useful clinical or research purpose.

CHAPTER 12
■Impulse Control Disorders

IN THIS CHAPTER:

- ■ Pathological Gambling
- ■ CAUTION: The Concept of Behavioral Addictions
- ■ Intermittent Explosive Disorder
- ■ CAUTION: Intermittent Explosive Disorder Diagnosis
- ■ Pyromania
- ■ Kleptomania
- ■ Unspecified Impulse Control Disorder
- ■ CAUTION: Avoiding Forensic Use of Unspecified Impulse Control Disorder

■ 312.31 PATHOLOGICAL GAMBLING

Screening Question

"How often do you gamble?"

Diagnostic Prototype

The gambling controls the person, rather than vice versa. He just can't get enough of it and has to keep raising the stakes to feel that old thrill ("tolerance"). Stopping causes withdrawal symptoms of irritability, restlessness, anxiety, and sadness, and the gambler can't wait to get more action ("withdrawal").

The person feels forced to continue gambling, despite the fact that it is no longer the fun it once was ("compulsive use"). She continues to gamble relentlessly, despite the terrible damage it keeps inflicting on finances, family, work performance, legal status, and self-respect.

CAUTION:
The Concept of Behavioral Addictions

DSM-5 accords Pathological Gambling the honor of its own section as the first Behavioral Addiction. In contrast, I have instead chosen to keep Pathological Gambling in its traditional place among the Impulse Control Disorders. The creation of a category especially for Behavioral Addictions is likely to open the Pandora's box of Unspecified Behavioral Addictions. I can picture this leading to the expansion of psychiatry to encompass a wide variety of life's pleasures and passions better left outside its purview—shopping, Internet surfing, video games, sex, exercise, collecting, sunbathing, and perhaps even model railroading. (For more detail, see the Caution box on this topic in Chapter 9.)

Differential Diagnosis:
Rule These Conditions Out

- **Recreational gambling.** The person still has fun gambling, is able to keep it under control, and doesn't get into serious trouble because of it.
- **Professional gambling.** The motive is profit, and the method is rational and carefully disciplined.
- **Manic Episode.** Gambling is an impulsive activity released during such an episode.

Diagnostic Tip

- **Relation to addictions.** The description of Pathological Gambling is closely modeled on the description of Substance Dependence. Both have a pattern of tolerance, withdrawal, compulsive use, and adverse consequences. What started out being recreational fun has now become a joyless preoccupation and compulsion.

■ 312.34 INTERMITTENT EXPLOSIVE DISORDER

Screening Question

"Do you ever become aggressive when you lose your temper?"

Diagnostic Prototype

The person has periods of uncontrolled angry outbursts that result in hurt people or destroyed property. The aggression is way out of line—much greater than makes sense, given whatever the provocation was.

Differential Diagnosis: Rule These Conditions Out

- **Another mental disorder.** Intermittent Explosive Disorder is a residual category only; it is not meant to be used if the aggressive behavior is an associated feature of any other mental disorder diagnosis.
- **A neurological disorder.** Refer the patient for an evaluation and testing.
- **Simple criminal behavior.** This is unrelated to a medical or psychiatric disorder.
- **Purposeful aggression.** The person is motivated by revenge or honor killing.
- **Normal anger of everyday life.** The outbursts do not cause clinically significant distress or impairment.
- **Malingering.** The person is trying to avoid facing the consequences of her actions.

Diagnostic Tips

- **Other mental disorders.** Aggressive behavior is not common, but can occur as part of many psychiatric episodes and disorders: Major Depressive Episodes, Manic Episodes, Schizophrenia, Substance Use Disorders, Delirium, Dementia, Antisocial Personality Disorder, Conduct Disorder, Borderline Personality Disorder, and others. When any of these disorders is present, it takes diagnostic priority, and a separate diagnosis of Intermittent Explosive Disorder is unnecessary.
- **The boundary between psychiatry and the law.** Intermittent Explosive Disorder may sometimes (probably very rarely) make sense as a diagnosis in mental health settings. It can never make sense in legal

proceedings as an excuse or exculpation for having committed harmful aggressive behavior.

CAUTION:
Intermittent Explosive Disorder Diagnosis

I am not convinced that Intermittent Explosive Disorder has merit as a mental disorder, and I doubt whether it should be included in DSM. Certainly the diagnosis should never be made until every other explanation has been carefully considered and ruled out. It is also inherently unreliable and not suitable for use in forensic proceedings. Estimates of its prevalence in epidemiological studies are likely to be meaningless.

■ 312.33 PYROMANIA

Pyromania has not been included in DSM-5, but it has an ICD-9-CM code and is clinically useful.

Screening Question

"Do you start fires?"

Diagnostic Prototype

The person loves everything about fires and gets great pleasure from starting them, watching them, helping to put them out, and watching what happens afterward.

Differential Diagnosis: Rule These Conditions Out

- **Arson for gain.** The aim of setting fire is to collect on insurance, not for the pure joy of it.
- **Arson as a political or terrorist act.**
- **Arson as a cover-up.** The person is destroying evidence of another crime.
- **Arson for vengeance.** The person has a vendetta and is acting in revenge.

- **Arson secondary to another mental disorder.**
- **Childhood experimentation.** Playing with fire has not yet established itself as a full pattern of Pyromania.

Diagnostic Tips

- **Avoiding overdiagnosis.** On careful evaluation, it turns out that most firesetting has other understandable motivations and should not be considered as evidence of mental disorder.
- **Other mental episodes and disorders in which firesetting occurs.** These include Intellectual Development Disorder, Delirium, Dementia, Substance Use Disorders, Schizophrenia, Manic Episodes, Antisocial Personality Disorder, and Conduct Disorder.

■ 312.32 KLEPTOMANIA

Kleptomania has also not been included in DSM-5, but it too still has an ICD-9-CM code and is clinically useful.

Screening Question

"Do you steal things?"

Diagnostic Prototype

People with Kleptomania steal things they don't really need for reasons they can't really explain, but they do get a kick out of doing it and feel relief afterward.

Differential Diagnosis: Rule These Conditions Out

- **Stealing for gain.** This accounts for the vast majority of shoplifters.
- **Stealing secondary to another mental disorder.**
- **Stealing due to substance-induced disinhibition.**
- **Stealing for vengeance.**
- **Teenage stealing.** The person is acting on a dare, in a group, for kicks, or to allay boredom.

Diagnostic Tip

• **Profit versus mental disorder.** Most shoplifters are in it for the goods, not for the kicks. In contrast, persons with Kleptomania take things they don't particularly want or need and often find ways to quickly dispose of them.

■ 312.30 UNSPECIFIED IMPULSE CONTROL DISORDER

CAUTION: Avoiding Forensic Misuse of Unspecified Impulse Control Disorder

The category of Unspecified Impulse Control Disorder is being misused in forensic situations. Don't be too free in using this category for every foolish thing that anyone does. There is a lot of impulsivity in this world, most of which is best not considered mental disorder. This is a residual and unreliable category not likely to have any meaning.

CHAPTER 13
■ Eating Disorders

IN THIS CHAPTER:

- ■ Anorexia Nervosa
- ■ Bulimia Nervosa
- ■ Binge-Eating Disorder
- ■ CAUTION: Binge-Eating Disorder
- ■ Unspecified Eating Disorder
- ■ CAUTION: Avoidant/Restrictive Food Intake Disorder

■ 307.1 ANOREXIA NERVOSA

Screening Question

"Do you feel fat, even though other people think you are way too thin?"

Diagnostic Prototype

She weighs very much less than she should, but still feels disgustingly fat. She is terrified of getting even fatter if she is not very careful about counting every calorie. She refuses to maintain a safe body weight, employing varying strategies like rigid dieting, excessive exercise, and purging by vomiting and laxatives. The weight loss is extreme—making her look like a concentration camp victim, and often endangering her health. Women stop having their period. Life is pretty much reduced to constant fretting about body image and frantic efforts to avoid anything that would help her gain much-needed weight.

Subtypes

- **Binge-Eating/Purging Type.** The weight loss and body image distortions are accompanied by binge eating and purging (vomiting, laxatives, diuretics, or enemas).
- **Restricting Type.** The person stays too thin just by diet and exercise.

Differential Diagnosis: Rule These Conditions Out

- **Bulimia Nervosa.** The person is normal-weight or overweight.
- **Weight loss caused by medical illness.** Examples of such illnesses include cancer and hyperthyroidism.
- **Weight loss caused by substance use.** An example is use of amphetamines.
- **Weight loss caused by another mental episode or disorder.** Examples include a Major Depressive Episode, a Manic Episode, or Psychotic Disorder.
- **Weight loss caused by poverty or bad eating habits.**
- **Normally thin frame and abstemious eating preferences.** There are no body image distortions and no dangerous weight loss.

Diagnostic Tips

- **Body image.** The key differentiating factors in the differential diagnosis are preoccupation with body image and the terror of becoming fat.
- **Medical exam.** Before making the diagnosis, a careful medical evaluation is necessary to ensure that the weight loss is not caused by a medical illness. After the diagnosis is made, careful medical monitoring is necessary to check for complications, since Anorexia Nervosa can have a high mortality rate.
- **Gender and cultural factors.** This diagnosis is much more common in females and occurs almost exclusively in developed, style-centered cultures.
- **Onset.** Usually in adolescence or early adulthood. Be cautious about making the diagnosis if the onset is later, and instead check carefully for medical causes.
- **Diet pills.** Evaluate whether the patient has a secondary Substance Dependence problem (e.g., using diet pills or amphetamine drugs).

■ 307.51 BULIMIA NERVOSA

Screening Question

"Do you often lose control and find yourself consuming a very large amount of food in a very short period of time?"

Diagnostic Prototype

She has periods of uncontrolled eating, with the consumption of really huge amounts of food. Then she tries to make up for the indulgence by compensatory actions like extreme fasting; exercising like crazy; or purging by vomiting, laxatives, enemas, or diuretics. The binges, the compensations for the binges, and their impact on body image become nagging preoccupations.

Subtypes

- **Purging.** The person uses vomiting, laxatives, enemas, or diuretics to compensate for binge eating. This subtype is more common and much more dangerous because purging can lead to many medical complications.
- **Nonpurging.** The person uses only exercise or fasting as compensations.

Differential Diagnosis: Rule These Conditions Out

- **Anorexia Nervosa.** The person has binges and purges, but is markedly underweight.
- **Binge-Eating Disorder.** There are no compensatory behaviors like purging, exercise, or fasting. See the Caution box on this disorder below, however.
- **Normal overindulgence.** There is no clinically significant distress or impairment.

Diagnostic Tips

- **Embarrassment.** People with Bulimia Nervosa tend to be terribly embarrassed about both the binge eating and the desperate things they do to compensate for it. You often have to get to know them very well and question them very closely before they will open up. Informants help.

- **Compensatory behaviors.** The diagnosis of Bulimia Nervosa requires compensatory behaviors. DSM-5 has introduced a new and controversial diagnosis, Binge-Eating Disorder, for patients who do the binge eating but without the compensatory behaviors. Again, for more on this, see the Caution box below.
- **Avoiding overdiagnosis.** From time to time, almost everyone binges and then tries to make up for it one way or the other. You should reserve this diagnosis for those who are doing it repeatedly, feel out of control, and are getting into trouble.
- **Binges versus grazing.** Binges are periodic, concentrated, and extraordinary "pig-outs." This is not the same as sustained, steady overeating. Obesity is not considered a mental disorder.
- **Occasional overindulgence.** Everyone will have an occasional overindulgence stimulated by holidays and "all you can eat" buffets. This doesn't count as a binge.
- **Diet pills.** As in Anorexia Nervosa, some people with Bulimia Nervosa develop a secondary Substance Dependence. Check for the use of diet pills or other substances to control weight.
- **Relation to Anorexia Nervosa.** People may oscillate back and forth between Anorexia Nervosa (Binge-Eating/Purging Type) and Bulimia Nervosa. Make the diagnosis appropriate for their current weight.

■ 307.51 BINGE-EATING DISORDER

Binge-Eating Disorder is one of the most controversial new diagnoses in DSM-5, and I recommend avoiding its use. See the Caution box below.

CAUTION: Binge-Eating Disorder

In DSM-5, Binge-Eating Disorder has been moved from the diagnoses included for further study to the main part (Section 2) of the manual. I worry that this diagnosis will be overused in everyday clinical practice, and I strongly advise against using it. Binge-Eating Disorder was created to diagnose people who have recurring eat-ing binges, without the compensatory activities like vomiting and laxative use seen in Bulimia Nervosa. The problem is that recurrent binge eating is a commonplace of human experience, not necessarily or usually a mental disorder. This diagnosis could easily become the most common in psychiatry, despite the fact that there has been very little research on how it should be defined and assessed, on its implica-tions for treatment, and on the risks and benefits of applying it to a given patient. In the rare clinical situation when this diagnosis seems needed, it can be coded as Unspecified Eating Disorder.

■ 307.50 UNSPECIFIED EATING DISORDER

Use Unspecified Eating Disorder when a diagnosis is definitely required for someone who does not meet the criteria for Anorexia Nervosa or Buli-mia Nervosa, but who still has clinically significant impairment. I also recommend using the Unspecified diagnosis not only for Binge-Eating Disorder (see the Caution box above), but for another controversial new diagnosis, Avoidant/Restrictive Food Intake Disorder (see the Caution box below).

CAUTION:
Avoidant/Restrictive Food Intake Disorder

DSM-5 has added Avoidant/Restrictive Food Intake Disorder to describe people who are particularly uninterested in eating or are restrictive or phobic in their food choices. They must also suffer resulting weight loss, nutritional deficiency, or social problems. There are two problems with this diagnosis: It merges into common and normal individual differences and preferences (e.g., fussy eating), and it has received far too little study to be qualified as an official mental disorder diagnosis. In the rare situation when it is needed, an Unspecified Eating Disorder code will suffice.

CHAPTER 14
■ Sleep–Wake Disorders

IN THIS CHAPTER:

- ■ Insomnia Disorder
- ■ Circadian Rhythm Sleep–Wake Disorder
- ■ Hypersomnolence Disorder
- ■ Sleep Apnea
- ■ Disorder of Arousal
- ■ Nightmare Disorder
- ■ Rapid Eye Movement Sleep Behavior Disorder
- ■ Substance-Induced Sleep–Wake Disorder
- ■ Insomnia Due to Another Medical Condition (Indicate the Medical Condition)
- ■ Hypersomnia Due to Another Medical Condition (Indicate the Medical Condition)
- ■ Unspecified Insomnia
- ■ Unspecified Hypersomnia

■ 307.42 INSOMNIA DISORDER

Screening Question

"Do you have trouble sleeping?"

Diagnostic Prototype

The person can't get enough satisfying sleep. There may be trouble falling asleep or waking up much too early, or choppy sleep in the middle of the night with lots of awakenings and endless tossing and turnings. The next day, the person feels irritable, tired, and sleepy, and is unable to think clearly. Work and relationships suffer. The person dreads the approach of bedtime and becomes increasingly convinced he will never, ever enjoy another good night's sleep.

Differential Diagnosis: Rule These Conditions Out

- **Normal "short sleeper" pattern.** Some people are lucky that way.
- **Patient who pushes to stay up.** The person could sleep more if she let herself.
- **Normally messed-up sleep.** This is the kind most of us have, especially if we don't allow enough time and relaxation to let nature take its course. It is an annoyance, certainly, but not a cause of clinically significant distress or impairment.
- **Problems with surroundings.** For example, the environment is noisy.
- **Poor sleep hygiene.** For example, the person takes excessive daytime naps, or exercises before bedtime.
- **Hypersomnolence Disorder.** Daytime sleepiness happens despite adequate nighttime sleep.
- **Circadian Rhythm Sleep–Wake Disorder.** The insomnia is related to sleeping out of sync.
- **Sleep Apnea.** Consider this diagnosis particularly in the elderly and obese.
- **Substance use or withdrawal.** This is a very common causal factor for insomnia.
- **Another mental disorder.** Insomnia is an associated symptom for so many mental disorders that it doesn't have to be coded separately unless it becomes particularly prominent and is the focus of special clinical attention.
- **A medical disorder.** Examples of such disorders include heart failure and hyperthyroidism.

Diagnostic Tips

- **Individual variability.** As in everything else in life, there is great human variety in sleep needs, and we have no clear standard to separate Insomnia Disorder from the run-of-the-mill sleep problems we all have.

- **Aging.** Like most skills, sleep deteriorates with age. It is unrealistic to expect to maintain the untroubled sleep of a babe throughout the life cycle. The standards for what is considered "normal" have to be adjusted for age.

- **Severity.** To be considered Insomnia Disorder, the sleep difficulty has to occur frequently and cause clinically significant misery and/or considerable impairment.

- **Duration.** Transient sleep problems are so common they don't count toward a diagnosis of Insomnia Disorder. The sleep problems must persist and pervade for many months.

- **Sleep hygiene.** Problems often improve with simple advice on how to develop healthier sleep habits.

- **Negative conditioning.** Vicious cycles develop when people become anxious about falling asleep and become negatively conditioned, especially to their own beds. Evidence of this: The person finds it easiest to sleep when away from the usual sleep environment (e.g., in a hotel room or another part of the house).

- **Substance use.** Never diagnose primary Insomnia Disorder until first ruling out the possible role of substances. Caffeine is the biggest culprit, but alcohol, recreational drugs, and prescription medicines are not far behind.

- **Sleeping pills.** Although these may help on any given night, their heavy, regular, and prolonged use may make Insomnia Disorder more severe and chronic.

- **Medical problems.** Illness can cause insomnia in different ways: by producing pain or discomfort; by a direct central effect on the brain (as in Delirium); or by general activation (as in hyperthyroidism). A medical examination is a useful part of the workup.

- **Sleep laboratory testing.** This may be warranted if the source of the Insomnia Disorder cannot be found and the sleep problems remain severe and persistent despite interventions. An interesting finding of such testing is that people generally sleep a lot better than they think they do.

■ 307.45 CIRCADIAN RHYTHM SLEEP–WAKE DISORDER

Screening Question

"Do you have a very irregular pattern of sleep?"

Diagnostic Prototype

The person can't fall asleep when he should and has trouble staying up when he must. Most commonly, this occurs in people who have to work the night shift or are always changing shifts, preventing the establishment of any regular sleep pattern. Circadian sleep problems also trouble those people whose work has them zipping through time zones faster than their brains can accommodate. Other people have such problems because of a disconnection between their internal clock and the demands of their world. "Night owls" love to stay up through the wee hours, but then may have trouble making it to work the next day. The "early birds" or "starlings" may drift off to sleep right over supper and then wake up in the middle of the night—all alone, but fully alert and raring to go. Some people, especially as they age, lose their previous capacity to maintain a regular rhythm of nighttime sleep.

Differential Diagnosis: Rule These Conditions Out

- **An irregular sleep pattern that is within normal limits.** The sleep pattern is not causing clinically significant distress or impairment.
- **Problems with surroundings or sleep hygiene.** There is a noisy environment, excessive daytime naps, or burning the midnight oil, for example.
- **Another Sleep–Wake Disorder.** Possibilities include Insomnia Disorder, Hypersomnolence Disorder, and Sleep Apnea.
- **Substance use or withdrawal.**
- **Another mental episode or disorder.** Examples include a Manic Episode, a Major Depressive Episode, and Schizophrenia.

Diagnostic Tips

- **Severity and duration.** This diagnosis shouldn't be given to someone who has a few days of jet lag. The broken sleep pattern must be severe and persistent, and must cause clinically significant distress or impairment.
- **Substance use.** Stimulants, especially if combined with "downers," can destroy sleep pattern—making day seem like night and night seem like day.

■ 307.44 HYPERSOMNOLENCE DISORDER

Screening Question

"Do you have to sleep more than most people?"

Diagnostic Prototype

The person gets 9 or 10 hours of sleep at night, but then still feels tired and needs naps during the day.

Differential Diagnosis: Rule These Conditions Out

- **"Burning the midnight oil."** Getting too little sleep at night is the most common cause of being tired during the day.
- **Naturally long sleep pattern.** These people have no clinically significant distress or impairment.
- **Insomnia Disorder or Circadian Rhythm Sleep–Wake Disorder.** The person is sleepy during the day because she is not able to get enough sleep at night.
- **A primary Depressive Disorder.** This can cause lethargy and increased need for sleep.
- **Substance use or withdrawal.** Examples include stimulant or caffeine withdrawal.
- **A medical illness.** Examples include hypothyroidism and brain tumor.

Diagnostic Tips

- **Individual variability.** Some people need more sleep than others, but function just fine otherwise and should get no diagnosis.
- **Gender differences.** Women tend to need more sleep than men.
- **Danger.** Hypersomnolence can be life-threatening, leading to car and other accidents. Advise the patient to reduce exposure to risky activities until the Hypersomnolence Disorder is under control.

■ 780.59 SLEEP APNEA

Screening Question

"Do you snore heavily, wake up a lot at night, and then feel tired during the day?"

Diagnostic Prototype

Some people with Sleep Apnea have prominent breathing difficulties during sleep, with loud snoring, gasping for breath, long periods without breaths, and frequent awakenings (sometimes with shortness of breath). Others with this disorder don't have the breathing dramatics, but do have the awakenings. Sleep Apnea is one cause of unrefreshing sleep and daytime sleepiness.

Differential Diagnosis: Rule These Conditions Out

- **Another current Sleep–Wake Disorder.**
- **A neurological or other medical disorder.**
- **Medication or other substance use.**

Diagnostic Tip

- **Status of Sleep Apnea.** Sleep Apnea is not a mental disorder. It is included here only because it is so often part of the differential diagnosis of Sleep–Wake Disorders. There are characteristic sleep laboratory findings that confirm the diagnosis.

■ 307.46 DISORDER OF AROUSAL

Screening Questions

For a parent: "Does your child walk or talk in her sleep or have sleep terrors?"

For an adult patient: "Have you been told that you walk or talk in your sleep or have sleep terrors?"

Diagnostic Prototype

Sleepwalking and sleep talking are most common in young children, who often eventually outgrow them. Usually these occur early in the nighttime sleep cycle and last only a few minutes; the children awake in the morning with no dreams or memory of the event.

Differential Diagnosis: Rule This Condition Out

- **Sleep arousals within normal limits.** These do not cause clinically significant distress or impairment.

Diagnostic Tip

- **Avoiding overdiagnosis.** Lots of kids have an occasional episode of sleepwalking or sleep talking that has absolutely no clinical meaning.

■ 307.47 NIGHTMARE DISORDER

Screening Question

"Do you suffer from nightmares?"

Diagnostic Prototype

The person has frequent and persistently terrible nightmares depicting awful life-threatening events. He wakes up vividly remembering the contents of the dream and fears falling asleep ("perchance to dream"). The nightmares usually occur during rapid eye movement (REM) sleep in the latter part of the nightly sleep cycle.

Differential Diagnosis: Rule These Conditions Out

- **The bad dreams we all have.** The nightmares must be frequent and persistent, and must cause serious sleep problems or impairment.
- **Sleep terrors.** These happen during non-REM sleep early in the sleep cycle, in a child who can't be easily awakened, who later has no remembered dream.
- **PTSD.** This takes diagnostic priority.
- **Another mental episode or disorder.** Examples include Delirium, a Manic Episode, and Panic Disorder.
- **Substance use.** For example, hallucinogens can cause nightmares.

Diagnostic Tips

- **Clinical significance.** There usually is none. In children, nightmares have little impact, and kids outgrow them spontaneously.
- **Secondary effects.** If there is clinical significance, it comes from the fear of falling asleep, insomnia, and the downstream consequences of this.

∎ 780.50 RAPID EYE MOVEMENT SLEEP BEHAVIOR DISORDER

Screening Question

"Have you been told that you do strange things while asleep?"

Diagnostic Prototype

The person doesn't have the usual sleep paralysis during REM sleep, enabling him to enact dreams with movements and vocalizations. Rarely, this may result in harming a bedmate. The episodes follow the pattern of REM activity—beginning 90 minutes after falling asleep, and occurring more commonly in the latter part of the night. On awakening, the person can usually report the dream or other aberrant behavior.

Differential Diagnosis:
Rule These Conditions Out

- **No diagnosis.** Disturbed behavior occurs during REM sleep, but no harm is done and it is not clinically significant.
- **Malingering.** The person uses REM Sleep Behavior Disorder as an excuse for spouse abuse.

Diagnostic Tip

- **Laboratory tests.** These may be necessary to confirm the diagnosis, particularly if there are forensic consequences.

▪ SUBSTANCE-INDUCED SLEEP–WAKE DISORDER

291.89 If Alcohol-Induced
292.89 If Induced by Any Other Substance (Indicate Substance)

Substance-Induced Sleep–Wake Disorder is an important part of the differential diagnosis for all of the primary sleep disorders. Virtually everyone who uses lots of substances has one or another problem with sleep, at least from time to time. This diagnosis is given only if the sleep problem is unusually prominent and has become the focus of clinical attention. It may be hard to distinguish Substance-Induced Sleep–Wake Disorder from Insomnia or Hypersomnia Due to Another Medical Condition (see below) in a patient who has a medical condition and takes medicine for it, both of which can disrupt sleep. Give both diagnoses when appropriate.

■ 780.52 INSOMNIA DUE TO ANOTHER MEDICAL CONDITION (INDICATE THE MEDICAL CONDITION)

■ 780.54 HYPERSOMNIA DUE TO ANOTHER MEDICAL CONDITION (INDICATE THE MEDICAL CONDITION)

Many sleep problems are caused by the effects of medical illness, either directly on the brain (as in Delirium) or because of pain and physical discomfort. Insomnia or Hypersomnia Due to Another Medical Condition is an important part of the differential diagnosis for all of the primary Sleep–Wake Disorders. A Medical Condition diagnosis is given only if the sleep problem is unusually prominent and has become the focus of clinical attention.

■ 780.52 UNSPECIFIED INSOMNIA

■ 780.54 UNSPECIFIED HYPERSOMNIA

Unspecified Insomnia or Unspecified Hypersomnia is a useful residual category for clinical presentations that are not clear-cut. More specific and accurate diagnosis may require sleep laboratory testing.

CHAPTER 15

■ Sexual and Gender Issues

IN THIS CHAPTER:

- ■ Gender Dysphoria
- ■ CAUTION: Gender Dysphoria
- ■ Sexual Dysfunctions
  - ● Male Hypoactive Sexual Desire Disorder
  - ● Erectile Disorder
  - ● Early Ejaculation
  - ● Delayed Ejaculation
  - ● Female Sexual Interest/Arousal Disorder
  - ● Female Orgasmic Disorder
  - ● Genito-Pelvic Pain/Penetration Disorder
  - ● Substance-Induced Sexual Dysfunction
  - ● Sexual Dysfunction Due to Another Medical Condition (Indicate the Medical Condition)
  - ● Unspecified Sexual Dysfunction
- ■ Paraphilic Disorders
  - ● Pedophilic Disorder
  - ● Exhibitionistic Disorder
  - ● Voyeuristic Disorder
  - ● Frotteuristic Disorder

- Sexual Sadism Disorder
- Sexual Masochism Disorder
- Fetishistic Disorder
- Transvestic Disorder
- Unspecified Paraphilic Disorder
- ■ CAUTION: Rejected Paraphilic Disorders

■ 302.XX GENDER DYSPHORIA

.6   Gender Dysphoria in Children
.85 Gender Dysphoria in Adolescents or Adults

CAUTION: Gender Dysphoria

Many clinicians and members of advocacy groups argue that issues related to gender choice should not be included at all in DSM-5—that gender choice is a matter of personal preference, not a mental disorder. I agree with them. But other clinicians and members of advocacy groups disagree; they make the reasonable argument that a code is sometimes necessary to support reimbursement for medical, surgical, and psychiatric treatment. There is no right answer, but one thing should be clear: The inclusion of Gender Dysphoria in DSM-5 does not imply that gender choice is by itself ever appropriate grounds for diagnosing a mental disorder.

Screening Question

"Do you feel that you were born in the body of the wrong gender?"

Diagnostic Prototype

The person has a cross-gender identification and discomfort living the life that usually goes with the anatomy the person was born with. This is manifested by persistent wishes to be the opposite sex, a rejection of the anatomy nature dealt, cross-dressing, and cross-gender role playing. In an adolescent or adult, there may also be efforts to change the external anatomy medically or surgically, to bring it into accord with the person's internal sense of self.

■ SEXUAL DYSFUNCTIONS

302.71 Male Hypoactive Sexual Desire Disorder

Screening Question

"Do you feel that your sexual desire is less than it should be?"

Diagnostic Prototype

He has little or no erotic fantasy life or sexual interest, and this causes distress or difficulty with partners.

Differential Diagnosis: Rule These Conditions Out

- **Sexual Dysfunction Due to Another Medical Condition.** The most obvious example of such a condition is testosterone deficiency.
- **Substance-Induced Sexual Dysfunction.** For example, alcohol, antihypertensives, and antidepressants can all cause low sexual desire.
- **A primary Depressive Disorder.** Low sexual desire occurs only during periods of low mood.
- **Partner Relational Problem.** The person lacks a stimulating partner, or there is psychological conflict with the partner. Use the appropriate V code (see Chapter 18).
- **Normal low sexual desire.**

Diagnostic Tips

- **Avoiding overdiagnosis.** There is great variation in what is considered normal, as well as great variability over the life cycle.
- **Mismatches.** Distress may arise out of a mismatch in sexual interest between the individual and his partner; it is useful to evaluate both partners.

607.84 Erectile Disorder

Screening Question

"Do you often have problems maintaining an erection?"

Diagnostic Prototype

He is unable to have an adequate erection during sexual activity, and this causes distress or difficulty with partners.

Differential Diagnosis: Rule These Conditions Out

- **Sexual Dysfunction Due to Another Medical Condition.** An example of such a condition is diabetes mellitus.
- **Substance-Induced Sexual Dysfunction.** For example, opiates can cause problems with erections.
- **Another mental disorder.** An example would be Major Depressive Disorder.
- **Partner Relational Problem.** The person lacks a stimulating partner, or there is psychological conflict with the partner. Use the appropriate V code.
- **Normal difficulty maintaining an erection.**

Diagnostic Tips

- **Avoiding overdiagnosis.** Again, there is great variation in what is considered normal, as well as great variability over the life cycle.
- **Mismatches.** Distress may arise out of a mismatch in sexual interest with his mate; it is useful to evaluate both partners.
- **The "Viagra effect."** Drug company hype for Viagra and similar medications can create unrealistic expectations.

302.75 Early Ejaculation

Screening Question

"Do you often ejaculate just after starting sexual activity?"

Diagnostic Prototype

He is repeatedly having a quick ejaculation after penetration, and this causes distress or difficulty with the partner.

Differential Diagnosis: Rule These Conditions Out

- **Substance-Induced Sexual Dysfunction.** The premature ejaculation is due to the direct effects of a substance (e.g., withdrawal from opiates).
- **Partner Relational Problem.** The person lacks a compatible partner, or there is psychological conflict with the partner. Again, use the appropriate V code.
- **Normal inexperience.**
- **No sexual activity in a long time.**

Diagnostic Tips

- **Avoiding overdiagnosis.** Once again, there is great variation in what is considered normal, and there is great variability over the life cycle.
- **Inexperience versus premature ejaculation.** Don't diagnose Early Ejaculation if someone has not yet had the opportunity to learn control.
- **Sex with a novel partner or after a long period of sexual abstinence.** Premature ejaculation is routine in these situations and is not a mental disorder. The premature ejaculation must be persistent and cause clinically significant impairments for Early Ejaculation to be diagnosed.

302.74 Delayed Ejaculation

Screening Question

"Does it take you too long to reach a climax during sexual activity?"

Diagnostic Prototype

He has delayed or absent ejaculation in most sexual encounters.

Differential Diagnosis: Rule These Conditions Out

- **Sexual Dysfunction Due to Another Medical Condition.** An example of such a condition is hyperprolactinemia.
- **Substance-Induced Sexual Dysfunction.** For example, alcohol and antidepressants can cause delayed or no ejaculation.

- **Another mental disorder.** For example, the orgasmic delay or absence occurs only during periods of depressed mood.
- **Partner Relational Problem.** He lacks a compatible partner, or there is psychological conflict with the partner. Again, use the appropriate V code.
- **Normal slow ejaculation, given age and situation.**

Diagnostic Tips

- **Avoiding overdiagnosis.** Once more, remember the wide range of normal. There must be clinically significant distress before Delayed Ejaculation can be diagnosed.
- **Making allowances for aging.** The time to ejaculation lengthens as one gets older.
- **Medication side effects.** For example, antidepressants and antihypertensives can cause this problem.

302.72 Female Sexual Interest/Arousal Disorder

Screening Question

"Do you feel that your sexual desire is lower than it should be, or that it is difficult for you to get sexually aroused?"

Diagnostic Prototype

She doesn't fantasize or have much interest in sex and has trouble getting aroused. This causes distress or problems with a partner.

Differential Diagnosis: Rule These Conditions Out

- **Sexual Dysfunction Due to Another Medical Condition.** Examples of such conditions include diabetes, lupus, and cancer.
- **Substance-Induced Sexual Dysfunction.** For example, antihypertensives and antidepressants can cause low desire.
- **A primary Depressive Disorder.** Low sexual desire occurs only during periods of low mood.

- **Partner Relational Problem.** She lacks a stimulating partner, or there is psychological conflict with the partner. Use the appropriate V code.
- **Normal low sexual interest.**

Diagnostic Tips

- **Avoiding overdiagnosis.** As emphasized above for men, there is great variation in what is considered normal, as well as great variability over the life cycle. An additional point to keep in mind for women is that drug companies are hyping Sexual Dysfunctions in women to sell pills.
- **Another "Viagra effect."** Distress may arise out of a mismatch in sexual interest with a mate who is suddenly more interested in sex because he is taking Viagra or a similar drug.

302.73 Female Orgasmic Disorder

Screening Question

"Do you usually find it hard to achieve climax during sex?"

Diagnostic Prototype

She can't reach a climax at all or it takes a very long time, and this causes distress or difficulty with a partner.

Differential Diagnosis:
Rule These Conditions Out

- **Sexual Dysfunction Due to Another Medical Condition.** An example of such a condition is diabetes mellitus.
- **Substance-Induced Sexual Dysfunction.** For example, antidepressants can cause difficulty with reaching orgasm.
- **Another mental disorder.** For example, Major Depression can result in orgasmic difficulty.
- **Partner Relational Problem.** She lacks a stimulating partner, or there is psychological conflict. Again, use the appropriate V code.
- **Normal trouble reaching a climax.**

Diagnostic Tips

- **Avoiding overdiagnosis.** Once again, there is great variation in what is considered normal, as well as great variability over the life cycle. Moreover, as noted above for Female Sexual Interest/Arousal Disorder, drug companies are hyping Sexual Dysfunctions in women to sell pills.
- **Context.** Does the woman lack sexual experience or a stimulating partner?
- **Another "Viagra effect," revisited.** Distress may arise out of a mismatch in sexual interest with a partner.

302.76 Genito-Pelvic Pain/Penetration Disorder

Screening Question

"Does vaginal intercourse usually hurt?"

Diagnostic Prototype

She has trouble allowing penetration because of pain or vaginal tensing.

Differential Diagnosis: Rule These Conditions Out

- **Sexual Dysfunction Due to Another Medical Condition.** An example of such a condition is a urinary tract infection.
- **Substance-Induced Sexual Dysfunction.** For example, estrogen antagonists can cause pain or tensing.
- **Somatic Symptom Disorder.** The pain is one of many somatic symptoms.
- **Partner Relational Problem.** For example, she lacks a stimulating partner or there is psychological conflict. Once more, use the appropriate V code.
- **Normal pain or discomfort.**

Diagnostic Tip

- **Severity and duration.** Do not use this diagnosis for mild pain, occasional pain, or pain due to lack of lubrication or rough sex.

Substance-Induced Sexual Dysfunction

291.89 If Alcohol-Induced
292.89 If Induced by Any Other Substance (Indicate Substance)

Screening Question

"Could alcohol or drug use have anything to do with your sexual problems?"

Diagnostic Prototype

The sexual symptoms are caused by a substance taken recreationally or by a prescribed medication.

Differential Diagnosis: Rule These Conditions Out

- **Another mental disorder.** The sexual disorder is incidental or unrelated to the substance or medication.
- **Substance Intoxication or Withdrawal.** The sexual symptoms are no greater in severity or longer in duration than those that occur in simple Substance Intoxication or Withdrawal.
- **Sexual Dysfunction Due to Another Medical Condition.** For example, hypothyroidism can cause sexual difficulty.
- **Normal substance-induced sexual problems.** The sexual problems are not a cause of clinically significant distress or impairment.
- **A primary Sexual Dysfunction.**

Diagnostic Tips

- **Medication side effect.** Many people take medicines that cause one or another form of sexual difficulty. Always do a careful history of medication use before assuming that a sexual disorder is primary. Antidepressants are particular offenders in this regard.
- **Chronology.** The substance or medication use should begin or increase before the onset of the sexual symptoms. Withdrawing the substance should, within a month or so, result in the disappearance or significant reduction of the symptoms.

- **Combined causes.** Sexual Dysfunction may be caused by a combination of medical or psychiatric illness and the medicines used to treat it. In such cases, diagnose both causal factors.

Sexual Dysfunction Due to Another Medical Condition (Indicate the Medical Condition)

608.89 Male Hypoactive Sexual Desire Disorder Due to Another Medical Condition

607.84 Erectile Disorder Due to Another Medical Condition

625.8 Sexual Interest/Arousal Disorder in Women Due to Another Medical Condition

625.0 Genito-Pelvic Pain/Penetration Disorder Due to Another Medical Condition

Specify the code depending on the type of Sexual Dysfunction caused by the medical condition.

Screening Question

"Did your sexual problem begin or get worse around the time you got sick or started taking a medicine?"

Diagnostic Prototype

The sexual symptoms are caused by the physical effects of a medical illness.

Differential Diagnosis: Rule These Conditions Out

- **A primary Sexual Dysfunction.** The substance use is incidental, unrelated, or secondary to the depression.
- **Substance Intoxication or Withdrawal.** The symptoms are no greater in severity or longer in duration than would be expected in simple Substance Intoxication or Withdrawal.
- **Normal sexual difficulty associated with illness.** It is not associated with clinically significant distress or impairment.

Diagnostic Tips

- **Chronology.** The medical illness should begin before the onset of the sexual symptoms, and improvements in the medical illness should result in the disappearance or significant reduction of the symptoms.
- **Age.** In older people, there should be an especially high index of suspicion that medical illness may be involved.
- **Medical examination and laboratory testing:** A thorough medical examination is indicated before it can be determined whether the Sexual Dysfunction is primary or is related to a medical condition.

302.70 Unspecified Sexual Dysfunction

The Unspecified Sexual Dysfunction diagnosis is particularly useful when it is unclear whether the Sexual Dysfunction is primary or results from substance use or a medical condition (or some combination).

■ PARAPHILIC DISORDERS

302.2 Pedophilic Disorder
302.4 Exhibitionistic Disorder
302.82 Voyeuristic Disorder
302.89 Frotteuristic Disorder
302.84 Sexual Sadism Disorder
302.83 Sexual Masochism Disorder
302.81 Fetishistic Disorder
302.3 Transvestic Disorder
302.9 Unspecified Paraphilic Disorder

Screening Question

"Do you have troubling sexual fantasies? Or have you ever gotten into trouble because of your sexual behavior?"

General Diagnostic Prototype for the Group

He has deviant sexual fantasies, urges, and behaviors that are persistent, are strong, and occur repeatedly. They are his preferred or required way of getting sexually excited, and he finds them distressing or they negatively affect his day-to-day life. There must also not be a better explanation for the behaviors (e.g., simple opportunistic criminality, disinhibition resulting from substance use, or poor judgment resulting from Intellectual Developmental Disorder or Schizophrenia). Paraphilic Disorders occur almost exclusively in men.

Specific Prototype for Each Paraphilic Disorder

The individual must meet the description above in one of the following ways.

302.2 Pedophilic Disorder

He prefers or requires sexual contact with prepubescent children for arousal. The person must be at least 16 years old and must be at least 5 years older than the child.

302.4 Exhibitionistic Disorder

He prefers or requires exposure of sex organs to strangers for arousal, perhaps combined with masturbation.

302.82 Voyeuristic Disorder

He prefers or requires peeping at strangers when they are having sex or disrobing, perhaps combined with masturbation.

302.89 Frotteuristic Disorder

He prefers or requires rubbing up against strangers in crowded places for arousal.

302.84 Sexual Sadism Disorder

He prefers or requires the infliction of pain or humiliation as a condition of sexual excitement.

302.83 Sexual Masochism Disorder

He prefers or requires receiving pain or humiliation as a condition of sexual excitement.

302.81 Fetishistic Disorder

He prefers or requires use of fetish objects (panties, bras, stockings, shoes) as a cue to sexual excitement.

302.3 Transvestic Disorder

He is a heterosexual male who prefers or requires cross-dressing as a means of becoming sexually excited.

302.9 Unspecified Paraphilic Disorder

See the diagnostic tips and the Caution box below for comments on the frequent misuse of Unspecified Paraphilic Disorder diagnoses in forensic evaluations.

Differential Diagnosis: Rule These Conditions Out for the Group

- **Behavior within limits of normal sexual arousal.**
- **Opportunistic criminal behavior.** The behavior is not preferred or obligatory (e.g., child victims are chosen because they were available and less able to put up a fight).
- **Disinhibition due to substance use.** The behavior occurs while the person is under the influence of a substance and is not preferred or obligatory.

- Disinhibition due to Intellectual Developmental Disorder.
- Disinhibition due to Dementia.
- Disinhibition due to a Manic Episode, Schizophrenia, or another mental episode or disorder.

Diagnostic Tips

- **The limits of "normal."** There is great variation in "normal" sexual practice. The definition of what is considered "deviant" versus what is considered acceptable in sexual behavior differs greatly over time and across cultures.
- **Potential for misuse.** Psychiatry should stay out of the bedroom or the court system unless there is a good reason for giving a mental disorder diagnosis.
- **Sexual deviance as an aspect of other conditions.** Occasional deviant sexual behaviors that are part of opportunistic crime, substance-induced disinhibition, another mental disorder, or Intellectual Developmental Disorder do not count toward a diagnosis of a Paraphilic Disorder.
- **Pedophilic Disorder.** It is important to restrict the Pedophilic Disorder diagnosis to men who have a recurrent, intense, obligatory need for prepubescent children as objects of sexual excitement. These men must be distinguished from simple criminals who opportunistically use children as sexual objects because they are vulnerable, or because adult partners are unavailable, or because they are under the disinhibiting influence of a substance. The emphasis is on establishing that a person specializes in kids because they are his preferred or obligatory sexual objects—not because they are vulnerable targets of opportunity. This crucial distinction has often been ignored in forensic evaluations.
- **Rape is a crime, not a mental disorder.** Unspecified Paraphilic Disorder, Nonconsent is a mostly fake and completely unreliable diagnosis created for forensic purposes. It has been widely misapplied to rapists to qualify them inappropriately for involuntary psychiatric commitment (in hearings conducted under "sexually violent predator" statutes). This ignores the fact that rape has been rejected as a mental disorder in DSM-III, DSM-III-R, DSM-IV, and DSM-5. Rape is almost always an

opportunistic behavior that reflects simple criminality—not a mental disorder. To establish that any given rapist also qualifies for a very rare Paraphilic Disorder diagnosis, it would be necessary to demonstrate that the use of force is necessary for him to become sexually excited, not (as is far more usual) that the force is just an incidental and instrumental means of gaining the victim's forced compliance and cooperation. It must also be shown that rape behavior is the man's preferred or obligatory means of achieving sexual excitement. And there would have to be a careful differential diagnosis that rules out far more common explanations: opportunistic rape; disinhibition due to substance use; revenge or anger rape; date rape; gang rape; and rape for profit (as with pimps). Unspecified Paraphilic Disorder, Nonconsent has been carelessly, unreliably, and incorrectly diagnosed in forensic hearings as a convenient way of promoting inappropriate psychiatric preventive detention. This is a misuse of psychiatric diagnosis and an abusive (and questionably constitutional) use of involuntary psychiatric commitment. Unspecified Paraphilic Disorder, Nonconsent should not be taken seriously when presented in expert testimony.

- **Sexual Sadism Disorder.** This diagnosis has also been misused in "sexually violent predator" hearings as an excuse for involuntary psychiatric commitment. This is an extremely rare disorder that is almost never encountered in clinical practice and has been described almost exclusively among serial murderers. It is not to be confused with the instrumental use of force, which is a routine and inherent part of all rapes. In Sexual Sadism Disorder, the man gets sexually excited by the act of inflicting pain or humiliation on the victim. Inflicting pain is the goal of the sexual act, not an incidental result of forcing compliance to gain cooperation. This must be the preferred or obligatory means of gaining excitement, and the sexual act is usually performed in a ritualized and stereotypic way to amplify the victim's suffering. Sexual Sadism must also be distinguished from the deliberate infliction of pain to express anger or to gain revenge, and also from occasional disinhibition caused by Substance Intoxication.

- **Unspecified Paraphilic Disorder diagnoses.** These are inherently unreliable and are therefore unsuitable in forensic proceedings. Unfortunately, Unspecified Paraphilia has been used widely and almost always inappropriately in involuntary commitment proceedings.

CAUTION: Rejected Paraphilic Disorders

The diagnosis of Paraphilia has been carelessly applied in hearings to determine involuntary psychiatric commitment for repeat sexual offenders under "sexually violent predator" statutes. Simple criminality is often confused with mental disorder. Although DSM-III, DSM-III-R, DSM-IV, and DSM-5 have all rejected the proposed diagnosis Paraphilic Coercive Disorder, it is still frequently but incorrectly offered to justify prolonged psychiatric commitment of rapists. This is an abuse of psychiatric diagnosis. DSM-5 also explicitly rejected the concept of Hebephilia (i.e., the proposal that it is a mental disorder to have sex with a postpubescent child). The concept of Hebephilia also has no place in forensic proceedings.

CHAPTER 16

■ Disorders Related to Physical Symptoms

IN THIS CHAPTER:

- ■ Somatic Symptom Disorder
- ■ CAUTION: Avoid Overdiagnosing DSM-5 Somatic Symptom Disorder
- ■ Conversion Disorder (Functional Neurological Symptom Disorder)
- ■ Psychological Factors Affecting Medical Condition
- ■ Factitious Disorder

■ 300.82 SOMATIC SYMPTOM DISORDER

DSM-5 has created the composite Somatic Symptom Disorder category (which now encompasses what were known in DSM-IV as Somatization Disorder, Hypochondriasis, Pain Disorder, and Undifferentiated Somatoform Disorder) for instances when concern about physical symptoms reaches the level of clinically significant distress or impairment. This new category is ridiculously overinclusive, and I recommend that it be used only when clearly needed (see the Caution box on pages 177–178).

Screening Question

"Are you consumed by worries about your health?"

Diagnostic Prototype

The person is completely preoccupied by bodily symptoms and/or health worries—well beyond what anyone would consider reasonable, and to a degree that causes clinically significant distress/impairment and clearly requires clinical attention. The preoccupation is severe, pervasive, persistent despite negative medical testing, resistant to realistic reassurance, and far out of line with any real health risk. Life has become so centered around health issues that daily rhythms, family, and work are severely compromised. Visits to doctors are frequent and frustrating; no one has any satisfying answers or constructive solutions.

Differential Diagnosis: Rule These Conditions Out

- **Everyday health concerns.** Everyone has these, but very rarely do they cause clinically significant distress or impairment that requires a diagnosis of mental disorder.
- **An undiscovered medical illness.** A medical disease may be causing the unexplained physical symptoms. Many conditions present with puzzling physical symptoms that take a while to cohere into a clear medical diagnosis. Don't assume that symptoms are psychological just because the diagnosis is still unclear. Uncertainty is hard to live with, but much better than jumping to false and risky conclusions.
- **Expectable reaction to having a medical illness.** This diagnosis should not be used for people who have cancer, diabetes, heart disease, or the like, and are vigilant and concerned about new symptoms that don't clearly fit the usual pattern for their illness. If any diagnosis is required, use Adjustment Disorder.
- **Another mental disorder.** Physical symptoms are common in Depressive, Bipolar, Anxiety, and Psychotic Disorders; Body Dysmorphic Disorder; and many other mental disorders.
- **Malingering.** Symptoms are consciously feigned or exaggerated for gain.
- **Factitious Disorder.** Symptoms are consciously feigned or exaggerated to acquire the advantages of the sick role.

Diagnostic Tips

- **A boundary puzzle.** These patients are at the boundary between psychiatry and medicine, present a daunting challenge to both, and are often handled well by neither. Close collaboration between medical personnel and mental health clinicians is essential.

- **Careful medical evaluation.** Don't quickly assume that the problem is necessarily in the patient's head. If symptoms are unexplained, it could be because previous medical workups were not thorough enough or because a medical illness has not yet sufficiently declared itself.

- **Avoiding overevaluation and excessive treatment.** Patients can accumulate an unbelievable amount of unnecessary medical testing and irrelevant treatment that are not only costly, but often actually dangerous to their health. The numerous doctors are often working at cross-purposes or duplicating each other's efforts. Try to centralize and coordinate diagnosis and care.

- **Evaluation for other mental disorders.** Somatic symptoms are often the first sign of a Bipolar, Depressive, Anxiety, or Psychotic Disorder, or some other mental disorder. Making a diagnosis in this section should be your last, not your first, choice and should come only after all pertinent mental and medical disorders have been ruled out.

- **Having some somatic symptoms as part of life.** An inevitable result of human anatomy and psychology is that we are troubled by unexplained and unexplainable bodily symptoms. These do not constitute a mental disorder unless they begin to have a serious impact on function, causing clinically significant distress or impairment.

- **Cultural factors.** In many parts of the world (and in Western countries until recently), somatic symptoms were the predominant means of expressing psychological distress. Different cultures have highly varying thresholds of acceptance of somatic symptoms as being normal and everyday versus being a sign of mental disorder. Clinical evaluation of somatic symptoms must be done within the context of the patient's cultural background.

CAUTION: Avoid Overdiagnosing DSM-5 Somatic Symptom Disorder

I recommend that clinicians be careful not to be overly inclusive in diagnosing DSM-5 Somatic Symptom Disorder. This diagnosis may mislabel medical problems as mental disorders (1) by encouraging a quick jump to the often erroneous conclusion that someone's physical symptoms or worries are "all in the head"; and (2) by mislabeling as mental disorders what are really just the normal emotional reactions that people understandably have in response to a medical illness.

The harms of inappropriate psychiatric diagnosis in the medically ill include stigma, loss of self-esteem, and negative perceptions by caregivers and family; missed medical and psychiatric diagnoses because of premature closure and incomplete workups; prescription of inappropriate psychotropic drugs; and disadvantages in employment, in medical and disability reimbursement, in provision of medical and social services, and in workplace accommodations.

The boundary between medical and psychiatric illness is inherently difficult to draw, especially since many psychiatric disorders do present with prominent somatic symptoms that are easily mistaken for medical illness. The best example is that people with panic attacks often get far too many medical tests for the dizziness, shortness of breath, and palpitations that are really just part of the hyperventilation caused by the panic attacks. And the emotional distress some people have in reaction to real or feared illness does sometimes get out of all proportion enough to require psychiatric attention. But there are serious risks attached to over-psychologizing somatic symptoms and mislabeling normal reactions to being sick.

■ 300.11 CONVERSION DISORDER (FUNCTIONAL NEUROLOGICAL SYMPTOM DISORDER)

Screening Question

"Do you ever get paralyzed or lose sensation or have fits?"

Diagnostic Prototype

The person has neurological symptoms that can't be explained after a thorough neurological workup. Most common are seizures, paralysis, gait disturbances, and difficulty with speech or swallowing. Very often, symptoms follow a stressful event, express a psychological conflict, or confer a secondary gain.

Differential Diagnosis: Rule These Conditions Out

- **A neurological illness.** For example, a person misdiagnosed with Conversion Disorder goes on to die of a brain tumor.
- **A primary Psychotic Disorder**. "Pseudohallucinations" in Conversion Disorder occur with intact reality testing, occur without other psychotic symptoms, involve multiple senses, and are unconvincing.

- **Malingering or Factitious Disorder.** The symptoms are consciously faked.

Diagnostic Tips

- **Atypical presentation.** Patients with Conversion Disorder often have symptoms that don't follow any anatomical pattern. The more sophisticated and experienced the patient, the closer will be the fit with neurological reality.
- **Relation to real illness.** The best mimics of a real disorder are those who actually have it (e.g., people with both Conversion Disorder seizures and real seizures).
- **Cultural factors.** Conversion Disorder was common in Western cultures until 100 years ago; now it has become quite rare. But in many other parts of the world (and in some parts of our world), Conversion Disorder remains one of the most frequent of presenting complaints.
- **Fads.** Conversion symptoms can be catchy, sometimes simultaneously affecting large numbers of people in episodes of "mass hysteria."

■ 316 PSYCHOLOGICAL FACTORS AFFECTING MEDICAL CONDITION

Screening Question

"Does your psychological state have an influence on how things are going with your medical illness?"

Diagnostic Prototype

The person's medical illness is made worse by psychological factors, which can be extremely varied. For example, Major Depression may increase risks after a heart attack; a passive–aggressive patient may not follow prescription instructions; someone in denial may refuse needed surgery; stress may predispose a patient to migraine headaches; a Christian Scientist may not seek medical care for asthma; or noncompliance with treatment may lead to a relapse of the medical illness.

Differential Diagnosis: Rule These Conditions Out

- **Mental Disorder Due to Another Medical Condition**. The medical condition adversely affects psychological health, rather than vice versa.
- **Factitious Disorder and Malingering**. The medical illness is feigned.

Diagnostic Tips

- **Not a mental disorder.** Psychological Factors Affecting Medical Condition is not considered to be a mental disorder and is included here only for purposes of convenience, to highlight problems that may contribute to medical illness or its treatment.
- **Factors adversely affecting medical illness.** These can include personality traits, stress, and an unhealthy diet and lifestyle.

■ FACTITIOUS DISORDER

300.16 Factitious Disorder With Psychological Symptoms

300.19 Factitious Disorder With Physical Symptoms

300.19 Factitious Disorder With Both Psychological and Physical Symptoms

Screening Question

"Are you making up or exaggerating any of your symptoms?"

Diagnostic Prototype

The person fakes being ill, psychologically or physically, to achieve the sick role and be taken care of. Being cared for as a perpetual patient has become a way of life. The person may drift from doctor to doctor and from hospital to hospital, with no other occupation and goal in life other than being a patient.

Differential Diagnosis: Rule These Conditions Out

- **Real illness**. The person is not faking it.
- **Malingering**. The person is faking it for a more understandable reason (e.g., to benefit financially or to avoid jail), not because she wants to be a patient receiving medical care.
- **Somatic Symptom Disorder**. Symptoms are not consciously faked.

Diagnostic Tips

- **Avoidance of overtesting and overtreating.** People with Factitious Disorder often become highly skilled at feigning a convincing clinical picture that can provoke extensive, expensive, redundant, and potentially extremely harmful diagnostic and therapeutic interventions.
- **Need for alertness to atypical or dramatic presentations of medical illness.** Those who are less skilled tend to overdramatize the sick role and have less command of the correct symptom presentations.
- **Need for alertness to real illness.** People with Factitious Disorder also get sick, often from the complications of previous medical interventions.

CHAPTER 17

■ Dissociative Disorders

IN THIS CHAPTER:

- ■ CAUTION: Dissociative Disorders—Fad Alert
- ■ Dissociative Identity Disorder (Multiple Personality Disorder)
- ■ CAUTION: Dissociative Identity Disorder (Multiple Personality Disorder)
- ■ Dissociative Amnesia
- ■ CAUTION: Dissociative Amnesia
- ■ Depersonalization/Derealization Disorder
- ■ Unspecified Dissociative Disorder

CAUTION: Dissociative Disorders—Fad Alert

The history of psychiatry has been filled with recurring fads of Dissociative Disorders. These take different forms. In this chapter, I provide cautions against two of them: Dissociative Identity Disorder (known until the publication of DSM-IV as Multiple Personality Disorder or MPD) and Dissociative Amnesia (fugue and recovered memories).

Fads in psychiatric diagnosis start with an exciting idea; a group of charismatic and gullible therapists then promotes it, and a growing army of suggestible and theatrical patients dramatizes and spreads it. "Dissociation" has often provided the exciting idea—in this case, the concept that something has been split off and repressed deep within a patient's psyche, and that she can be healed once it is returned to consciousness. The problem is that allegedly "repressed" material can take fantastic forms, shaped by the joint creative imaginations of the therapist and patient. What emerges from their efforts often bears little or no relation to either psychic reality or real reality.

■ 300.14 DISSOCIATIVE IDENTITY DISORDER (MULTIPLE PERSONALITY DISORDER)

Dissociative Identity Disorder, or MPD as I call it here, has been one of the most fad-prone of all the psychiatric diagnoses. It is dormant now, but steer clear of it when the next fad starts. **In fact, I recommend avoiding this diagnosis altogether.** In the Caution box below, I explain why.

CAUTION: Dissociative Identity Disorder (Multiple Personality Disorder)

Iatrogenesis

MPD almost always has its roots in enthusiastic therapists eliciting multiple personalities in highly suggestible patients.

Kindling the Fad

Often a hit movie or a best-selling book makes MPD a popular conversation piece. *The Three Faces of Eve* and *Sybil* made for good box office, but caused no end of mischief.

The Most Recent False Epidemic

The spread of MPD in the 1990s was promoted by poorly trained therapists encouraging their submissive and imaginative patients to get in touch with inner "alter" selves. Sometimes using hypnosis or other regressive techniques, they were able magically to transform inner psychological distress and conflict into previously "repressed personalities" who were somehow waiting to spring to life when summoned by these therapists.

The Profit Motive

MPD actually became something of a cottage industry. Numerous weekend workshops were held all around the country to train therapists in the exciting new techniques, which in fact were as old as a shaman's tool kit. After just a few days, newly minted "experts" on dissociation were turned loose to create new "alters" or "multiples." Long-term and expensive inpatient units were established to provide the perfect environment for multiplying personalities. And the Internet amplified it all, with patients supporting each other's multiplications in an almost competitive endeavor to see who could be divided into the most parts. I once saw a patient who claimed to contain within herself no fewer than 162 distinct personalities, of all ages and both sexes, in a constant chattering internal dialogue.

The Quick End of the Fad

The jig was up at about the turn of the century, when insurance companies stopped paying the bills. Patients magically brought together their divided parts and went on living as they had before the fad started. (A similar fad of MPD occurred in the late 19th century, when hypnosis was all the rage in Paris and Vienna. This fad ended equally abruptly when psychoanalysis replaced hypnosis as a favored treatment.)

The Moral of the Story

The moral of the story is this: **Don't follow fashionable fad diagnoses.** If everyone seems to have a new and suddenly popular diagnosis, then it is probably a mirage—and no one really has it. Should MPD make another comeback at some point in the future (as it undoubtedly will), don't be swept along by the hype. And please don't ever go to a weekend workshop on how to elicit "multiples."

What to Say to a Patient

A friend of mine had the best response to a patient who wanted to do nothing in sessions but create more personalities: "I don't care which of your personalities I talk to, so long as it is the one that wants to get better."

■ 300.12 DISSOCIATIVE AMNESIA

Screening Question

"Are there parts of your life you can't remember?"

Diagnostic Prototype

The person has "blank spots" in which personal memories, especially for events that were painful and stressful, are missing. Theoretically, there are two types of Dissociative Amnesia:

Simple amnesia: The person forgets specific things.

Fugue: The person supposedly forgets who he was and takes on a new identity.

CAUTION: Dissociative Amnesia

Fugue

Although the loss of an old identity and the taking on of a new one seem to happen all the time in the movies, I have never seen an actual case of fugue and don't think you will either. The theme seems to be endlessly intriguing, but I wonder whether true fugues ever really happen.

Recovered Memories

Twenty years ago, there was a fad of Dissociative Amnesia: People everywhere were suddenly recovering what turned out to be false memories. Under the tutelage of eager and poorly trained therapists, patients discovered that they had been raped as children by their parents; by other family members; or by teachers, caregivers, or sometimes even aliens. Childhood sexual abuse is a serious problem, but the sudden explosion of reports, their occurrence in a charged and suggestible "therapeutic" environment, and the bizarre implausibility of most of the stories suggest that Dissociative Amnesia was wildly overdiagnosed. The cost in family discord was high, and some parents and caregivers were prosecuted and even imprisoned on the flimsiest and most absurd evidence. This is another sad example of the potentially tragic consequences of fad-based overdiagnosis.

Differential Diagnosis: Rule These Conditions Out

- **Normal forgetting.** This happens all the time, especially as we age.
- **A neurological injury or disease.** For example, amnesia may be a result of head trauma.
- **Substance Intoxication or side effects of prescription drugs.** Both of these can cause blackouts.
- **PTSD or Acute Stress Disorder.** The memory loss is restricted to the stressful event.
- **Malingering.** "Forgetting" results in gain or the reduction of personal responsibility.

Diagnostic Tips

- **Normal forgetting.** Most people have only the patchiest of memories for most of their lives. Forgetting is commonplace; Dissociative Amnesia is vanishingly rare.
- **Residual nature of the diagnosis.** Other much more likely and treatable explanations of serious forgetting have to be carefully considered and ruled out.
- **Rarity of the diagnosis.** Blackouts are routine features of Substance Intoxication. Dissociative Amnesia is an exotic plant that you may not see in your entire career. As I have advised in Chapter 1 in regard to any rare diagnosis, "When you hear hoofbeats on Broadway, think horses, not zebras!"
- **Head trauma.** Any amnestic episode that occurs after a car accident is much more likely to be due to concussion than to the psychological trauma. And overlooking head trauma can be deadly.
- **"Letting sleeping dogs lie."** Remembering a terrible event is not always such a great thing or good idea. There is no reason to diagnose Dissociative Amnesia unless the forgetting is causing clinically significant distress or impairment. Many naïve therapists incorrectly assume that repression is always pathological. They may cause iatrogenic harm by not "letting sleeping dogs lie."

■ 300.6 DEPERSONALIZATION/DEREALIZATION DISORDER

Screening Questions

For depersonalization: "Do you ever get the weird detached feeling that you are watching yourself go through the motions of life?"

For derealization: "Do things ever seem unreal—like you are living in a dream world or in a movie even when you are awake?"

Diagnostic Prototype

Lots of us occasionally have the uncanny feeling of losing touch with ourselves. Instead of spontaneously just living life, it feels as if we are watching a stranger do what we do. We catch a glimpse of ourselves in the mirror and momentarily wonder, "Who is that person, and how am I connected to him [or her]?" This "depersonalization" is often accompanied by "derealization": The world suddenly loses its immediacy and plausibility, and instead seems weirdly out of joint—like a movie being run at the wrong speed. These experiences usually have no clinical significance. They often occur in young people as part of growing up and ebb gradually with age. To constitute a mental disorder, the depersonalization/derealization must be persistent and pervasive; must cause lots of distress or impairment; and must also stand alone and not be part of another condition.

Differential Diagnosis: Rule These Conditions Out

- **Normal depersonalization/derealization.** The symptoms don't have much of an impact on the person's life.
- **Substance Intoxication.** Intoxication with substances is by far the most likely cause of depersonalization/derealization.
- **Head trauma or other neurological condition.** For example, seizures can cause depersonalization or derealization.
- **Another mental disorder.** Just about every condition in psychiatry can cause depersonalization/derealization.

Diagnostic Tips

- **Depersonalization and derealization as symptoms rather than a diagnosis.** They rarely stand alone in a severe enough form to constitute a separate mental disorder.
- **Normality of depersonalization/derealization.** Difficulty feeling fully comfortable in one's own skin is a commonplace part of growing up. Only rarely does depersonalization or derealization constitute a mental disorder.
- **Reality testing.** For a diagnosis of Depersonalization/Derealization Disorder to be made, the person must still be in touch with reality.

Depersonalization/derealization can occur at a delusional level (i.e., patients actually believe that they are not themselves and/or that the world is unreal). This is a symptom of Schizophrenia or other Psychotic Disorders, or of severe Bipolar or Depressive Disorder with psychotic symptoms.

- **Residual nature of the diagnosis.** Depersonalization can be an associated symptom of most psychiatric disorders and also of various insults to the brain. Depersonalization/Derealization Disorder is to be diagnosed only when every possible specific cause has been ruled out.

- **Substance Intoxication.** As noted above, intoxication with various substances commonly causes or exacerbates depersonalization/derealization.

- **Frightening symptoms.** Some people (particularly those who have the symptoms during panic attacks) take depersonalization and/or derealization as a sign they are going crazy. Reassurance and normalization can be very helpful.

■ 300.15 UNSPECIFIED DISSOCIATIVE DISORDER

Certain culture-bound syndromes that include trance states may be diagnosed as Unspecified Dissociative Disorder if there is clinically significant distress or impairment.

CHAPTER 18

■ Codes for Conditions That May Be a Focus of Clinical Attention but Are Not Mental Disorders

■ INVITATION: PLEASE USE THESE CODES MORE OFTEN

A separate section of DSM-5 includes a number of commonly encountered situations that are explicitly not mental disorders, but nonetheless call for the special skills of mental health practitioners. There would be less diagnostic inflation in psychiatry (and the world would therefore be a better place) if the codes in this section were used more often and the codes for the various mental disorders were used less often. These codes are dramatically underused, in large part because insurance companies are often reluctant to reimburse for them—a policy that is not only clinically damaging, but shortsighted even on financial grounds. Once an unnecessary diagnosis is given, it takes on a life of its own and is likely to increase the person's overall lifetime utilization of services. It would be cheaper and more efficient to automatically cover brief episodes of service for these problems. It is also far better for people having expectable life problems to receive brief counseling teaching them coping skills to deal with the specific problems, instead of loading them with the misleading, confusing, and potentially harmful baggage of an unnecessary diagnosis of mental disorder.

■ RELATIONAL PROBLEMS

Mental disorders by definition occur only in individuals. Most problems requiring couple and family therapy are more accurately coded here.

V61.9   Relational Problem Related to a Mental Disorder or General Medical Condition

V61.20 Parent–Child Relational Problem

V61.10 Partner Relational Problem

V61.8   Sibling Relational Problem

V62.81 Unspecified Relational Problem

■ PROBLEMS RELATED TO ABUSE OR NEGLECT

Most aggressive behavior is not due to a mental disorder and should therefore be coded here. Likewise, most sexual abuse is not due to a mental disorder and should be coded here.

V61.21 Physical Abuse of Child
        (code 995.54 if focus is on victim)

V61.21 Sexual Abuse of Child
        (code 995.53 if focus is on victim)

V61.21 Neglect of Child
        (code 995.52 if focus is on victim)

V61.12 Physical Abuse of Adult (if by partner)

V62.83 Physical Abuse of Adult (if by person other than partner)
        (code 995.81 if focus is on victim)

V61.12 Sexual Abuse of an Adult (if by partner)

V62.83 Sexual Abuse of an Adult (if by person other than partner)
        (code 995.83 if focus is on victim)

■ MEDICATION-INDUCED MOVEMENT DISORDERS

332.1   Neuroleptic-Induced Parkinsonism

333.92 Neuroleptic Malignant Syndrome

333.7   Neuroleptic-Induced Acute Dystonia

333.99 Neuroleptic-Induced Acute Akathisia

333.82 Neuroleptic-Induced Tardive Dyskinesia

333.1   Medication-Induced Postural Tremor

333.90 Unspecified Medication-Induced Movement Disorder

■ OTHER PROBLEMS

V15.81 Noncompliance With Treatment

Noncompliance is a very important factor in treatment nonresponse.

V65.2   Malingering

Malingering needs to be considered in the differential diagnosis for many mental disorders.

V71.01 Adult Antisocial Behavior

Use Adult Antisocial Behavior when there is no history of Conduct Disorder.

V71.02 Child or Adolescent Antisocial Behavior

Use Child or Adolescent Antisocial Behavior when isolated misbehavior is not part of a pattern of Conduct Disorder.

V62.89 Borderline Intellectual Functioning

An IQ above 70 is not considered a mental disorder.

780.9 Age-Related Cognitive Decline

Age-Related Cognitive Decline is in the differential diagnosis for Major Neurocognitive Disorder (Dementia). Normal aging is not considered a mental disorder, although it may be causing the person's problems.

V62.82 Bereavement

Bereavement is definitely not a mental disorder. Major Depression should not be overdiagnosed when someone has the expectable symptoms of loss. This code should be used when a bereaved person needs clinical attention but is not mentally ill. Major Depression should be diagnosed only when symptoms are severe, suicidal ideation is prominent, or there are delusions.

V62.3 **Academic Problem**

V62.2 **Occupational Problem**

313.82 **Identity Problem**

V62.89 **Religious or Spiritual Problem**

V62.4 **Acculturation Problem**

V62.89 **Phase of Life Problem**

995.2 **Unspecified Adverse Effects of Medication**

■ Index of Disorders by Symptoms

■ M

Mania
Bipolar Disorder Due to Another
Medical Condition, 59
Bipolar I Disorder, 50–51
Delirium, 121–122
Substance Use Disorders, 112,
114–115, 116, 117, 118
Substance-Induced Bipolar
Disorder, 58
Unspecified Bipolar Disorder, 60
Memory Impairment
Acute Stress Disorder, 91
Bipolar I Disorder, 50–51
Bipolar II Disorder, 54–55
Delirium, 121–122
Dissociative Amnesia, 184–185
Major Depressive Disorder, 37–39
Major Neurocognitive Disorder
(Dementia), 125–126
Posttraumatic Stress Disorder, 88–89
Substance Use Disorders, 112,
114–115, 116, 117, 118
Mood swings
Bipolar I Disorder, 50–51
Bipolar II Disorder, 54–55
Cyclothymic Disorder, 57
Delirium, 121–122
Schizoaffective Disorder, 101–102
Motor behaviors
Autism Spectrum Disorder, 25–26
Medication-Induced Movement
Disorders, 191
Obsessive–Compulsive Disorder,
76–78
Tic Disorders, 85

■ N

Nightmares
Acute Stress Disorder, 91
Nightmare Disorder, 155–156
Posttraumatic Stress Disorder,
88–89

Noncompliance with treatment, V
code, 191

■ O

Obsessions
Anorexia Nervosa, 144
Body Dysmorphic Disorder, 81
Obsessive–Compulsive Disorder,
76–78
Obsessive–Compulsive or Related
Disorder Due to Another Medical
Condition, 87
Substance-Induced Obsessive–
Compulsive or Related Disorder,
86
Unspecified Obsessive–Compulsive
or Related Disorder, 87

■ P

Paranoia
Bipolar I Disorder, Severe With
Psychotic Features, 50–51
Bipolar II Disorder, Depressed,
Severe With Psychotic Features,
54–55
Brief Psychotic Disorder, 104–105
Delirium, 121–122
Delusional Disorder, 101–102
Major Depressive Disorder, Severe
with Psychotic Features, 38
Major Neurocognitive Disorder
(Dementia), 125–126
Paranoid Personality Disorder, 133
Psychotic Disorder Due to Another
Medical Condition, 107
Schizoaffective Disorder, 101–102
Schizophrenia, 95
Schizophreniform Disorder, 99–100
Schizotypal Personality Disorder, 134
Shared Psychotic Disorder, 104
Substance Use Disorders, 112,
114–115, 116, 117, 118